MW00490137

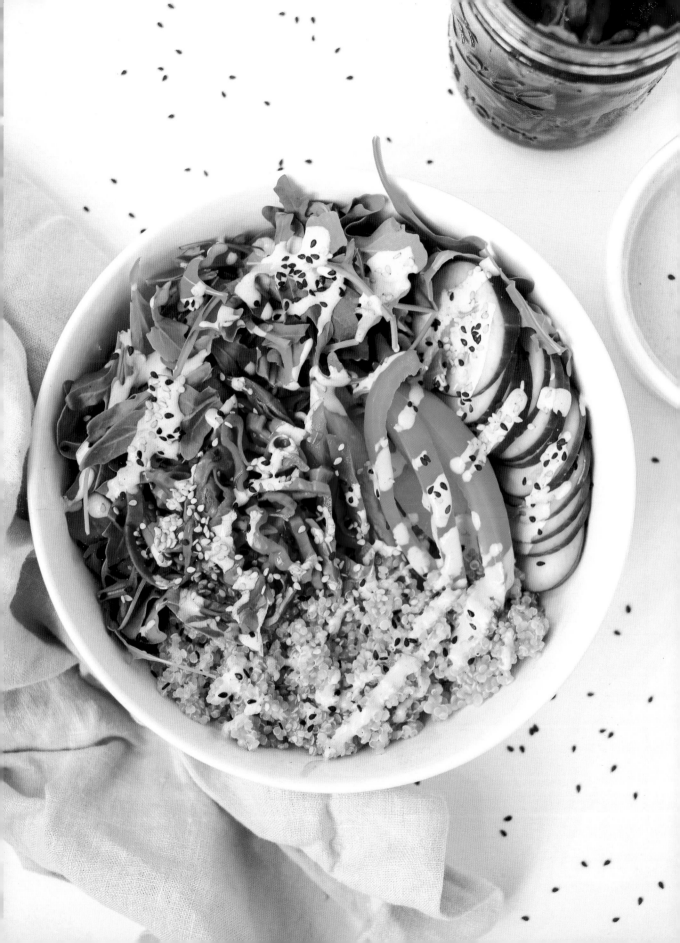

THE
Plant-Based
Cookbook
FOR WOMEN

Simple, Healthy Recipes to Increase Energy
and Balance Hormones

Shannon Leparski

CERTIFIED HORMONE SPECIALIST AND
AUTHOR OF *THE HAPPY HORMONE GUIDE*

BLUE·STAR
PRESS

BLUE·STAR
PRESS

Copyright © 2021 Shannon Leparski

Published by Blue Star Press
PO Box 8835, Bend, OR 97708
contact@bluestarpress.com
www.bluestarpress.com

All rights reserved. No part of this publication may be reproduced or transmitted in any form or by any means, electronic or mechanical, including photocopy, recording, or any information storage and retrieval system, without permission in writing from the publisher.

Design by Amy Sly
Food photography by Shannon Leparski
Author photos by Sara Hilton

ISBN: 9781950968183

Printed in Mexico

10 9 8 7 6 5 4 3 2 1

DISCLAIMER:
This book is for informational and educational purposes. The author is not a physician or medical professional. The information presented herein has not been evaluated by the U.S. Food and Drug Administration, and it is not intended to diagnose, treat, cure, or prevent any disease. Please consult your health-care provider before beginning or modifying any diet, exercise, or health-care program.

Dedication

For my happy hormone girls,
this cookbook is for you.

You gotta nourish to flourish.

Honor your hormones, be your own health
advocate, and never stop learning.

TABLE OF
Contents

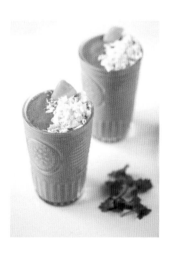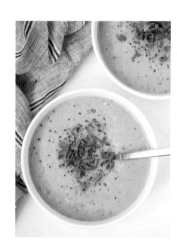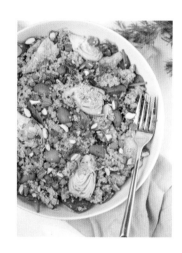

Menstrual Phase Recipes

Follicular Phase Recipes

Ovulatory Phase Recipes

Luteal Phase Recipes

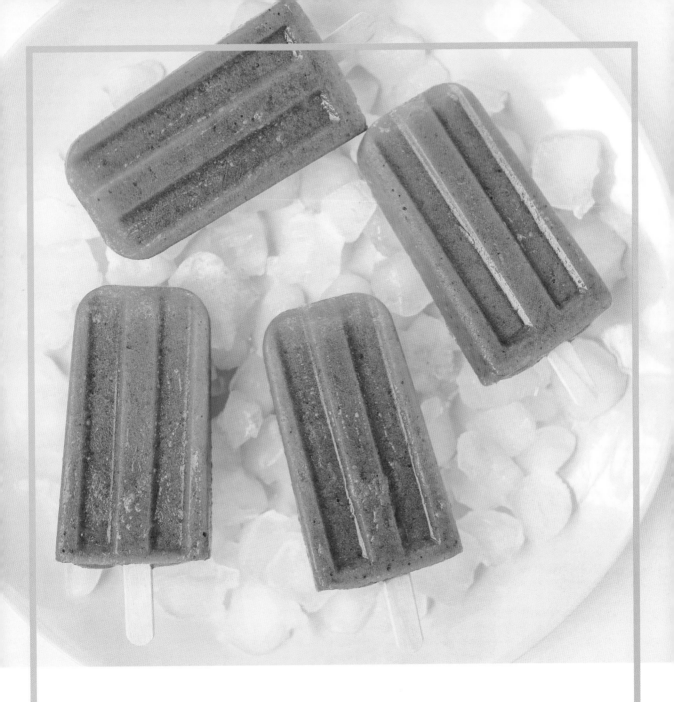

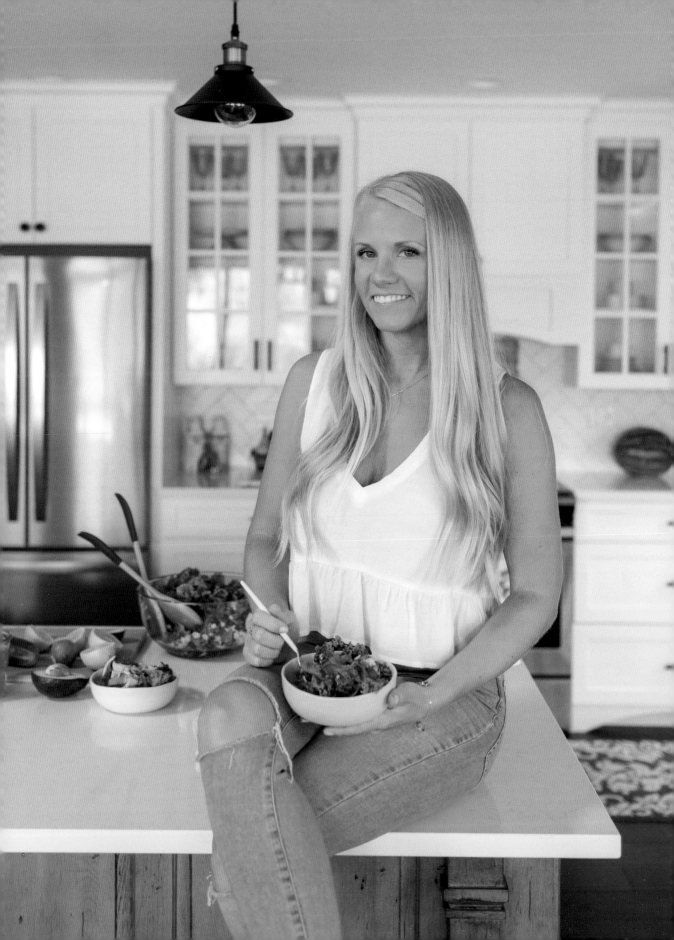

Introduction

What you eat has an enormous impact on your body, how you look and feel, your hormone function, and your overall health. In this sense, plant foods are a girl's best friend.

A plant-based diet can revolutionize your life. It can help balance your hormones, greatly reduce your risk for certain cancers, heart disease, and diabetes, and prevent or slow cognitive decline. It can also strengthen your immunity, beautify your skin, enhance digestion, increase fertility, and reduce your carbon footprint. Plain and simple: the more plants you eat, the better your health will be. Need I say more!?

Plant foods are a girl's best friend.

As a woman, your physical and emotional needs fluctuate as you naturally flow through your hormonal cycle each month. *The Plant-Based Cookbook for Women* is a guide to eating in tune with the four phases of your cycle—the menstrual, follicular, ovulatory, and luteal phases—so that you can strengthen your awareness of your body and work with your flow, not against it.

The phases of your cycle affect so much: how you feel, what you crave, the nutrients you need, how productive or motivated you are, the type of exercises you should do, your mood, your fertility, and more. Getting in sync with these fluctuations is a transformative act of self-care. This book promotes eating a variety of high-vibrational whole plant foods and makes it easy for you to consume the array of micronutrients that nutritionally support your hormonal fluctuations. Eating this way will help you naturally balance your hormones, allowing you to connect deeply to your body's inner wisdom, give it what it needs, and recognize your internal cues.

Plant-based nutrition is NOT about feeling deprived, counting calories, or portioning out your meals. It is not low calorie, low carb, low fat, or lacking in nutrients. It IS about nourishing your body with real, delicious, vibrant, rainbow-colored foods from the earth. It's about releasing yourself from diet culture and society's mandated ways of eating to discover what foods best support your body at certain times throughout your cycle. It is about honoring your hunger cues,

> # " Health will always start with the food on your plate. "

tuning into your needs, and eating to satisfaction. Plant-based eating gives you the freedom and power to heal your body from the inside out. Health will always start with the food on your plate.

My first book, *The Happy Hormone Guide,* presented an in-depth lifestyle program called "The Happy Hormone Method" for syncing up with the phases of your cycle—including phase-friendly workouts, DIY skin and hair treatments, supplements, herbs, essential oils, seed cycling, nutrition, and more. Since what you eat is such a huge part of hormone function, I saw an opportunity to provide even more recipes to help women tune into their bodies through plant-based foods. In this cookbook, you'll find 80 delicious recipes for breakfast, lunch, dinner, dessert, and snacks—20 for each of the four phases of your cycle.

I also explain how to create a meal plan using a mix-and-match approach to the recipes in the book, if that appeals to you. I want you to choose the recipes that feel best for you; I'm not interested in telling you what to eat and when! Remember, this approach to nutrition is about freedom, liberation, and satisfaction. Every day is different, and you are not a robot! I recommend starting by picking four or five recipes to make each week and seeing how it goes. Slowly rotate through all of the recipes in this book and notice what feels best for you. I've included plenty of options so that you can use this cookbook for a long time and always come back to it. And if you're craving more, I have hundreds of recipes on my blog, "The Glowing Fridge," categorized into the four phases of the cycle.

The Hundred–Day Journey

What you do today will affect your hormones in three months. Mind-blowing, right? I refer to this as The Hundred-Day Journey. This basically means that when you start eating healthy, nutrient-rich, plant-based foods for your cycle, you are putting coins in the bank for your hormones, health, and skin three months from now. It also means that you want to give your body at least three months to see improvements from this new way of eating. Change doesn't happen overnight, but when it happens, you'll know because you will be radiating from the inside out.

So, why three months? It takes 100 days for a follicle to develop from its inactive state and become mature enough for ovulation. A healthy cycle requires healthy follicles. What you did three months ago affects your cycle today. Take a moment to think back to three months ago. Were you super stressed? Did you move or change jobs? Did you go through a break-up or a major life change? Were you drinking more or eating more junk food than usual? All of these factors affect the health of your follicles over the course of 100 days. I love shining light on this topic because we often don't connect the dots in this way.

Here's what you may notice after just three months of following the recipes in this cookbook:

- Clearer and brighter skin
- Improved sleep
- Increased energy
- Better and more stabilized mood
- Fewer PMS symptoms
- Ovulation regularity
- Increased libido
- Enhanced digestion

Getting To Know Your Cycle Phases

Before we dive into the recipes, here is a quick primer on the phases of your cycle. Just like the lunar moon cycle, your body transitions through your four phases every 28-30 days, on average. To learn more about each phase, your endocrine system, toxins, and more, check out *The Happy Hormone Guide*! The more you know, the more you'll be able to tune into your body's unique needs.

Let's take a quick look.

MENSTRUAL PHASE
Winter, New Moon (lasts 3-7 days)

The menstrual phase is the bleeding phase and is known as the "winter" season in your body. Consider it a chance to rest, conserve energy, and hibernate. It is said to be a time when there is little distinction between intuition and logic, allowing you to gain deeper access to your inner wisdom and gut feelings. The bleeding phase is naturally cleansing (physically and emotionally), so while you may feel raw and sensitive, remember that you are also letting go of what no longer serves you.

If you do not become pregnant, then 12 to 14 days after ovulation, the corpus luteum (what is left of the follicle after the egg was released) stops making progesterone and gets reabsorbed in your body. This drop in progesterone is what triggers your uterus to contract and start your bleed. Day one of your period begins on the first day of heavy bleeding—not just light spotting. This is great information to know for tracking purposes.

During this phase, hormones are at very low levels, which means you may have lower energy, your skin may look somewhat dry and dull, and you may feel more run-down than usual. This is generally the time to take it easy. It's also the time to focus on replenishing lost minerals and restoring your blood with foods rich in the nutrients iron, zinc, and iodine. Foods like Swiss chard, kale, kidney beans, tofu, tempeh, seaweeds, kelp, edamame, beets, beet greens, mushrooms, and pumpkin seeds will be particularly nourishing.

FOLLICULAR PHASE
Spring, Waxing Moon (lasts 7-10 days)

The follicular phase is considered the "spring" season in your body. It begins after your period ends and brings a sense of growth, renewal, and productivity—and an urge to plan. You may be able to see a clear path ahead as life feels fresh and optimistic (which can be a nice change of pace after menstruation!).

This is the time when your body prepares to release an egg (which happens in the ovulatory phase). Each ovary has hundreds of thousands of follicles (sacs of cells containing an immature egg at the center). In the follicular phase, the pituitary gland is signaled to release FSH (follicle-stimulating hormone) to stimulate a number of follicles to grow (but only one will win and ovulate!). The maturing follicles release the hormone estradiol to thicken the uterine lining for implantation, should the egg become fertilized.

This phase is all about increased energy, an awakened libido, elevated mood, and creativity. Because your brain chemistry is optimized at this time, planning out your life feels like a breeze! Proper nutrients are essential for your maturing follicles to be healthy enough for ovulation. Eat fresh, colorful foods that are higher in fat and rich in potassium, vitamin A, vitamin B6, and vitamin C, as well as probiotic-rich foods. Think about incorporating avocado, spinach, carrots, broccoli sprouts, asparagus, green peas, olives, citrus, cherries, plums, pomegranate, tofu, lentils, mung beans, ground flaxseed, cashew butter, and pumpkin seeds during this phase. Think of it as your spring—a time of new beginnings and trying new things.

Change doesn't happen overnight, but when it happens, you'll know.

> Understanding why you're having certain symptoms at certain times will empower you to combat them in healthy ways.

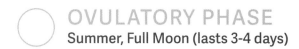 OVULATORY PHASE
Summer, Full Moon (lasts 3-4 days)

The ovulatory phase is known as the "summer" season in your body. Life flows somewhat effortlessly in this phase. You feel playful, flirty, and more outgoing than usual. You are MAGNETIC, which is ideal because this is when you are at your peak of feeling your most beautiful! This phase is all about having fun, connecting with others, and allowing yourself to embrace getting a little more attention than usual.

Ovulation is the main event of your cycle. Typically, you are only fertile for 24 hours in your cycle (when the egg is released), but sperm can live inside you for up to 5-7 days (I know, right?). That's because your fertile cervical mucus nourishes the sperm and keeps it alive. Understanding when you are ovulating allows you to avoid intercourse, use protection, or time intercourse—depending on the outcome you're after.

Around day 12 of your cycle, the dominant follicle secretes a big surge of estrogen, prompting a flood of luteinizing hormone (LH). This causes the dominant follicle to grow rapidly until around day 14 (but varies for each woman) when the follicle finally ruptures and releases the egg. This is why you may feel a sharp twinge or cramping on one or both sides of your abdomen when you ovulate. Ovulation is a vital part of the menstrual cycle and is the only way your body is able to make progesterone in the next phase (the luteal phase).

During this phase, your skin may look extra glowy, the whites of your eyes may appear brighter, you may feel more social and talkative, and you'll have lots of energy and a high libido. The ovulatory phase is the perfect time to enjoy and thrive on tropical raw fruits and veggies. Their nutrients will help keep things moving and increase your levels of the antioxidant glutathione, which is important for liver detoxification to assist your body in eliminating estrogen. Glutathione can be found in high-fiber whole foods and liver-detoxifying (bitter) foods like dandelion greens, turmeric, sprouts (of any kind), and milk thistle tea. Raw green juices are also great during this phase, as well as big veggie salads and vegetable soups.

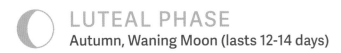

LUTEAL PHASE
Autumn, Waning Moon (lasts 12-14 days)

The luteal phase is known as the "autumn" season in your body. This is a time to turn inward, reflect, and gain clarity. It's also a time to prep for "winter" and get things done that you've been putting off all month. You may feel inclined to finish projects, clean out your closet, meal prep, or deep clean the house. This is all thanks to progesterone, the calming, anti-anxiety hormone that regulates your mood and promotes deep sleep.

In order to make progesterone, you must ovulate. The corpus luteum (what's left of the follicle after the egg was released) forms into an endocrine gland and starts making progesterone. This is meant to maintain and nourish a pregnancy, should a fertilized egg be implanted. If not, the corpus luteum gets reabsorbed, progesterone plummets, and you get your period! It's an AMAZING process.

The luteal phase is also when PMS may strike. The hormonal fluctuations may make your skin break out. Lower estrogen levels also mean less collagen, so your skin may feel less plump or glowy. It's a good time to focus on grounding and nourishing foods that are high in magnesium and vitamin B6 like roasted root vegetables, yams, and ginger. Eating complex carbohydrates that are high in fiber like chickpeas, squash, parsnips, and pumpkin will also help combat sugar cravings, which can deter mood swings. Understanding *why* you're having certain symptoms at certain times will empower you to combat them in healthy ways. That's the magic of eating for your cycle!

Simple Meal Planning

Strict meal planning is a thing of the past—it doesn't take into account your fluctuating hormones, individual appetite, or overall lifestyle. I just can't get behind a one-size-fits-all approach to healthy living. Nourishing your body is all about knowing your options and having good food and ingredients readily available in your home. Buying your own groceries and making your own food saves you money; plus, plant-based food is much cheaper than processed or boxed foods.

Here is my version of meal planning: I usually make two grocery trips a week. I make one trip early in the week on Sunday or Monday, and another later in the week to stock up for the weekend. Figure out a schedule that works for you and try to stick to it. When I know that I have beautiful plant-based food in my fridge, I'm inspired to make something out of it, or else it's a total waste! The trick is to make a loose plan of what you want to cook over the next few days, make a list of the items you need, and stick to it. A grocery trip without a list usually ends with me forgetting something and having to go back (or worse, buying a bunch of random things I won't end up eating!).

Meal planning is a form of self-care. To meal plan with this book, first think about what phase you'll be in for the upcoming week. Flip to that section and see which recipes appeal to you and what you'll need to make each recipe over the coming days. This process eliminates the pressure of constantly worrying about what your next meal will be because it's already (loosely) planned out. Plus, you'll have the

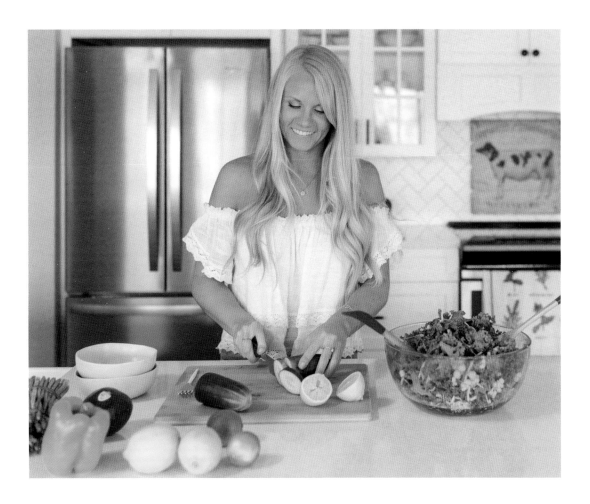

comfort of knowing that your plan aligns with your body's needs for that cycle phase.

In this book, you'll find 20 recipes for each phase of the cycle, so you have plenty of options! Depending on how your week looks, pick out 4-5 recipes and make a grocery list using them. When you get home from the store, wash your produce, prep what you can for your next couple of meals (in terms of sauces, grains, beans, or whatever you can easily make ahead) and properly store your ingredients, so they are ready to go. This makes eating healthy all week long a total breeze! The minimal time you spend prepping and shopping is a gift to your future self.

Stocking Your Kitchen

The recipes in this book are intentionally simple and accessible to anyone. You don't need a bunch of fancy kitchen gear or expensive ingredients to get started. In my plant-based journey, I've come across a few tools and go-to ingredients that can make this lifestyle easier. Here are some of my favorites. Find what works for you!

Tools And Supplies:

You don't need to run out and purchase all of these tools, but the items in this list will help make healthy cooking easier for you! Having good tools in your kitchen makes all the difference.

- **NutriBullet:** I use my NutriBullet more than any other kitchen tool. I love it for single-serving smoothies, grinding flaxseeds, and making sauces like pesto or queso. I like how the NutriBullet is small, has different sized cups, and is super powerful. It's also inexpensive and a great option for cooking for one or two people.

- **High-Speed Blender:** If you have a family, I would invest in a high-speed blender like a Vitamix or Blendtec. I use mine when I'm blending two or more servings of a smoothie, for blending soups, and for making larger portions of sauces (like a mac and cheese sauce, or something I want to store in the freezer for later use). A high-speed blender will give you that restaurant-quality smoothness, especially if you are sensitive to texture.

- **Hand Immersion Blender:** A hand immersion blender comes in handy for soups, especially when you don't feel like transferring the hot liquid from a pot to a blender. You can just blend directly in the pot! It won't provide as smooth of a texture as a high-speed blender, but sometimes I prefer this with soups when I want to leave in some chunks of potatoes or beans. It's also much easier to clean up than a blender or NutriBullet.

- **Food Processor:** Many of the recipes in this cookbook call for a food processor, so you'll want to get your hands on one if you don't already have one in your kitchen. Food processors are for shredding vegetables, grinding nuts and seeds,

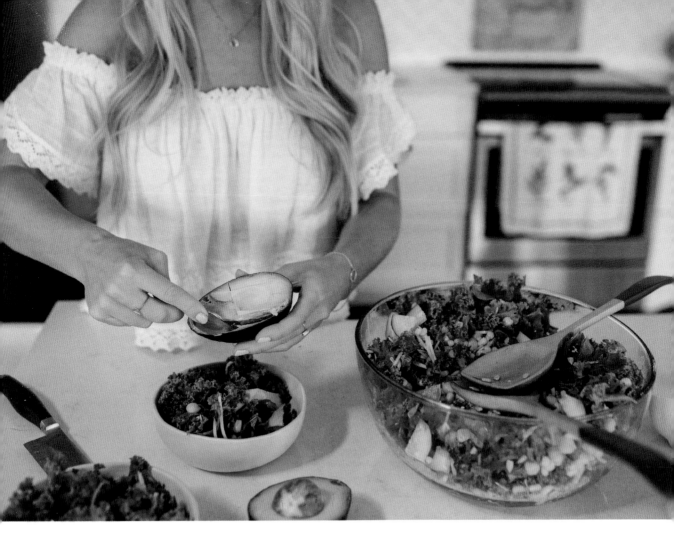

turning oats into oat flour, mixing dough, or making things like pesto. I have a Cuisinart 10-cup food processor, which seems to be the perfect size for most recipes. If you get a smaller one, you may have to work in batches, whereas, with a bigger one, you'll have to stop and scrape down the sides more. There are plenty of sizes and options to work for all budgets.

- **Non-Toxic Pots and Pans:** Nonstick cookware is often coated with the chemicals PFTE (polytetrafluoroethylene) or PFOA (perfluorooctanoic acid), which have been linked to a host of health conditions. They are one of the main reasons I wish people would reconsider the cookware they use. I like Green Pans and highly recommend them. Using unhealthy cookware to cook healthy food just doesn't make sense. While I know it may be a burden to replace all of your cookware, carrying the burden of toxins associated with cancers, hormone disruption, and other serious health problems is a much greater weight. I promise you'll get lots of great use out of your healthy pots and pans with all of the recipes you'll be making from this cookbook!

- **Wooden Utensils:** I suggest stocking up on wooden utensils like serving spoons and spatulas instead of metal, as these can scrape the bottom of your pots and pans.

- **Bamboo or Non-Toxic Cutting Boards:** Stay away from plastic cutting boards if possible since they are often coated in chemicals. Natural materials are preferred for food prep.

- **Salad Scissors:** These aren't necessary, but they are relatively inexpensive and a fun and easy way to make restaurant-quality chopped salads.

- **Mandoline Slicer:** This simple tool makes it easy to thinly slice vegetables.

- **Spiralizer:** A spiral vegetable slicer is a great tool for whenever you want to get creative and make "noodles" out of your favorite vegetables like zucchini or carrots.

- **Mason Jars:** I love having a bunch on hand in different sizes. They're great for serving smoothies and storing sauces or dry goods.

- **Tofu Press:** A tofu press isn't a must, but it is a helpful tool for removing excess water, which helps create crispier tofu when cooking.

- **Mesh Strainer or Nut Milk Bag:** These come in handy when you are rinsing tiny grains like amaranth, or when you are making your own vegan cheese at home and need to remove small chunks of cashews from your mixture while cooking.

- **Water Filter:** I like to used filtered water in all my recipes to ensure I'm eating as clean as possible. Use the filter on your refrigerator or faucet, or get a filtered pitcher.

- **Airtight Storage Containers:** It's always useful to have a variety of different-sized storage containers in your kitchen for leftovers. I recommend containers made of glass because they are more sustainable and better for reheating than plastic.

Go-To Ingredients:

These are the things that I like to keep stocked in my pantry at all times. Whenever I run out of something, I put it on my grocery list so I can immediately restock. This way produce makes up the bulk of my grocery shopping, and I can rest assured that I already have the seasonings and other essentials I need waiting for me at home.

- **Grains:** brown rice, black rice, wild rice, quinoa, millet, rolled oats, rice noodles, buckwheat noodles

- **Legumes:** lentils, canned beans of all varieties, chickpea pasta

- **Canned/Packaged Goods:** low-sodium vegetable broth, crushed and diced tomatoes, green chiles, jarred roasted red peppers, sun-dried tomatoes

- **Flours:** almond flour, coconut flour, oat flour, tapioca flour/starch, gluten-free flour blend

- **Oils:** coconut oil, avocado oil, olive oil, sesame oil

- **Chocolate:** cacao powder, cacao nibs, vegan chocolate chips

- **Coconut:** shredded coconut, canned coconut milk, coconut water

- **Nuts and Seeds:** walnuts, cashews, almonds, brazil nuts, pecans, peanuts, pistachios, flaxseeds, pumpkin seeds, sesame seeds, sunflower seeds, hemp seeds, chia seeds

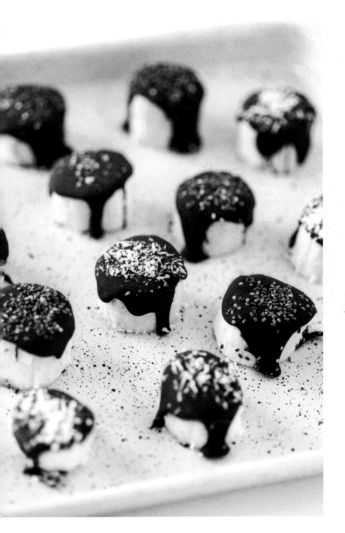

- **Nut and Seed Butters (raw and unsweetened):** almond butter, peanut butter, cashew butter, sunflower seed butter, tahini

- **Sweeteners:** Stevia liquid drops, pure maple syrup, coconut sugar, medjool dates, raisins

- **Condiments:** Apple cider vinegar, Dijon mustard

- **Spices and Flavorings:** tamari, nutritional yeast, sea salt, kala namak (black salt), black pepper, crushed red pepper flakes, cinnamon, chili powder, paprika, cumin, turmeric, ginger, oregano, thyme

- **Refrigerator:** tofu, tempeh, raw sauerkraut, sprouts

- **Freezer:** frozen bananas, frozen berries and other frozen fruit, gluten-free bread, corn or Siete brand tortillas, shelled edamame, frozen peas, frozen organic corn

Menstrual Phase

Your menstrual phase, also known as the "winter" season of your cycle, is the time to focus on replenishing minerals and restoring your blood and kidneys with nutrient-rich foods. Your body is doing a lot of internal work right now, including eliminating the lining of your uterus! Foods rich in iron and zinc will be particularly nourishing, so try to consume mushrooms, Swiss chard, kale, kelp, beets, beet greens, tofu, tempeh, black beans, kidney beans, pumpkin seeds, and blackstrap molasses. Cook with sea salt and tamari and utilize lots of sea vegetables to help refresh trace minerals. Sea vegetables are also especially high in iodine, which plays an important role in thyroid health and breast health. Use cooking methods that feel natural and easy (not stressful!) during this phase since it is a time to rest and conserve energy. Think about cooking warming and comforting soups and stews like the Rustic Potato, Kale, and Kidney Bean Stew or the simple Crispy Tofu and Buckwheat Noodle Stir-Fry. When you're in the mood for something refreshing, try smoothies with dark berries, kale, and flax like the Ultimate Period Smoothie, or snack on watermelon or grapes. Other foods that will provide an added boost for the menstrual phase include hazelnuts, wild rice, seaweeds, chlorophyll, adzuki beans, and coconut water.

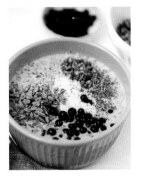

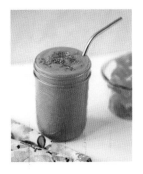
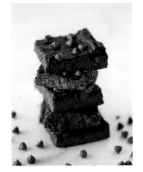

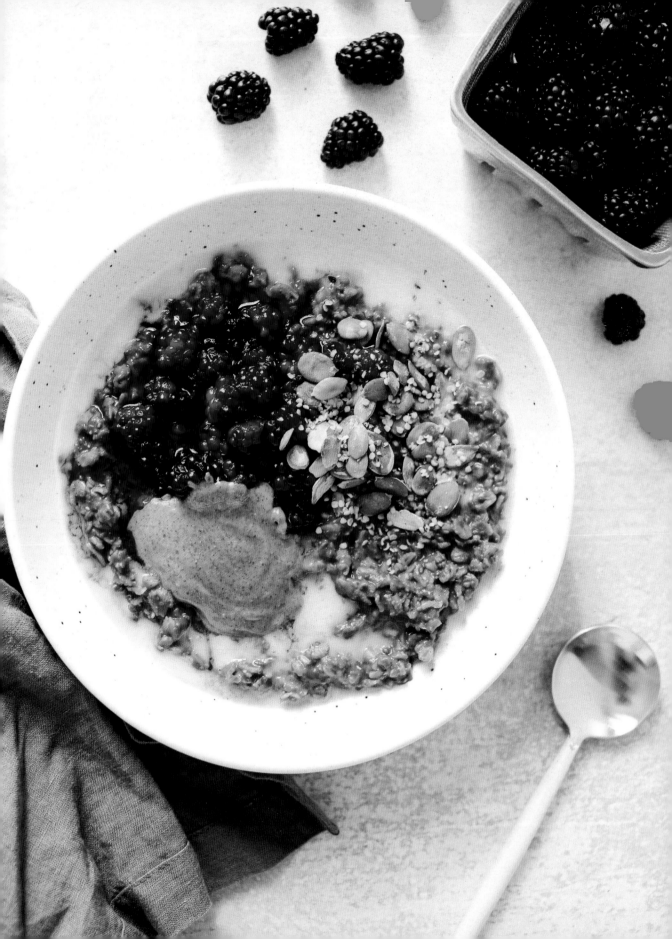

Prep Time: 5 minutes   **Cook Time:** 25 minutes   **Total Time:** 30 minutes

Blackberry Compote Chocolate Oatmeal

Level up your morning with a bowl of this decadent gluten-free warming oatmeal! It's comforting (with a hint of sweetness) and feels just right during your period. It has a chocolate taste from the cacao powder, but the blackberry compote is what really steals the show. To cut down on the sugar, I combined liquid stevia and pure maple syrup. Add toppings of your choosing for some added texture and nourishment.

Combine the oats, coconut milk, and water in a medium saucepan over medium-high heat. Bring to a boil, then reduce the heat to simmer. Stir in the cacao powder, chia seeds, liquid stevia, vanilla extract, and sea salt. Cover and let simmer, stirring occasionally, for 10–15 minutes.

Meanwhile, combine all the ingredients for the blackberry compote in a smaller saucepan over medium heat. Stir well. Bring to a slow boil, then reduce the heat and let simmer for 5–7 minutes, until the sauce has reduced.

Divide the oatmeal between two bowls and layer the blackberry compote on top. Add the optional toppings and an extra splash of coconut milk for creaminess and serve. Store leftovers in an airtight container in the refrigerator for up to 3 days.

SERVES: 2

OATMEAL

1 cup gluten-free rolled oats

1 cup coconut milk (or any plant-based milk), plus more if needed

1 cup filtered water

2 tablespoons raw cacao powder

1 tablespoon chia seeds

2 dropperfuls liquid stevia (or 1 tablespoon monk fruit sugar or pure maple syrup)

½ teaspoon vanilla extract

Pinch of sea salt

Optional toppings: ground flaxseed, pepitas, hemp seeds, almond butter

BLACKBERRY COMPOTE

6 ounces (or 3/4 cup) blackberries, halved

1 tablespoon pure maple syrup

1 tablespoon almond butter

½ teaspoon ground cinnamon

Mushrooms on Toast

SERVES: 2

2 tablespoons coconut oil
(or vegan butter)

8 ounces (or 1 cup) baby bella
mushrooms, sliced (or any other kind
of mushroom)

1 clove garlic, minced

½ teaspoon onion powder

½ teaspoon black pepper

¼ teaspoon sea salt

1 ½ teaspoons red wine vinegar

4 slices thick gluten-free bread

1 large ripe avocado, mashed

Optional toppings: dulse flakes,
red pepper flakes, everything
bagel seasoning

Treat yourself to a fancy version of classic avocado toast. The savory, hearty mushrooms offer the extra plant protein and immune boost you need during your period, while also satisfying your cravings. This is one of my go-to breakfast recipes because it's simple and comes together quickly. I like to serve the toast with a side of fruit—think watermelon, grapes, or berries during this phase—or a fresh green juice (preferably with beets).

Heat a frying pan over medium-high heat and add the coconut oil. Once the oil is melted and the pan is hot, add the mushrooms and cook, stirring constantly until lightly browned, 5–7 minutes. Add the garlic, onion powder, black pepper, sea salt, and red wine vinegar and stir to coat. Continue to sauté for 2 more minutes. Meanwhile, toast the bread slices until golden. Spread each slice with avocado, then spoon 3-4 tablespoons of mushrooms over the top. Sprinkle with the optional toppings, then serve two slices of toast on each plate. Store any leftover mushrooms in an airtight container in the refrigerator for up to 2 days.

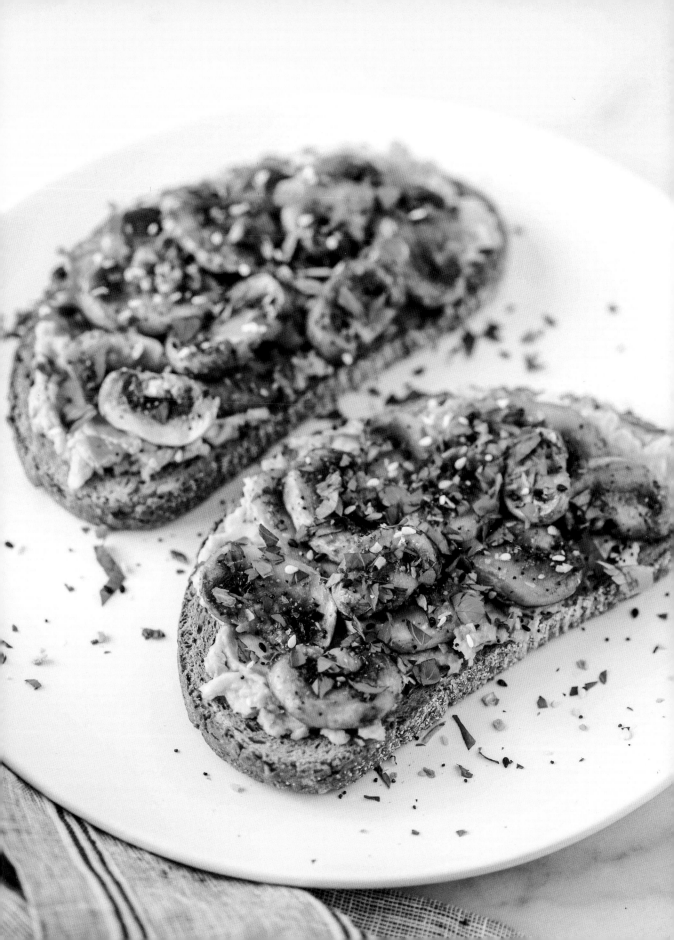

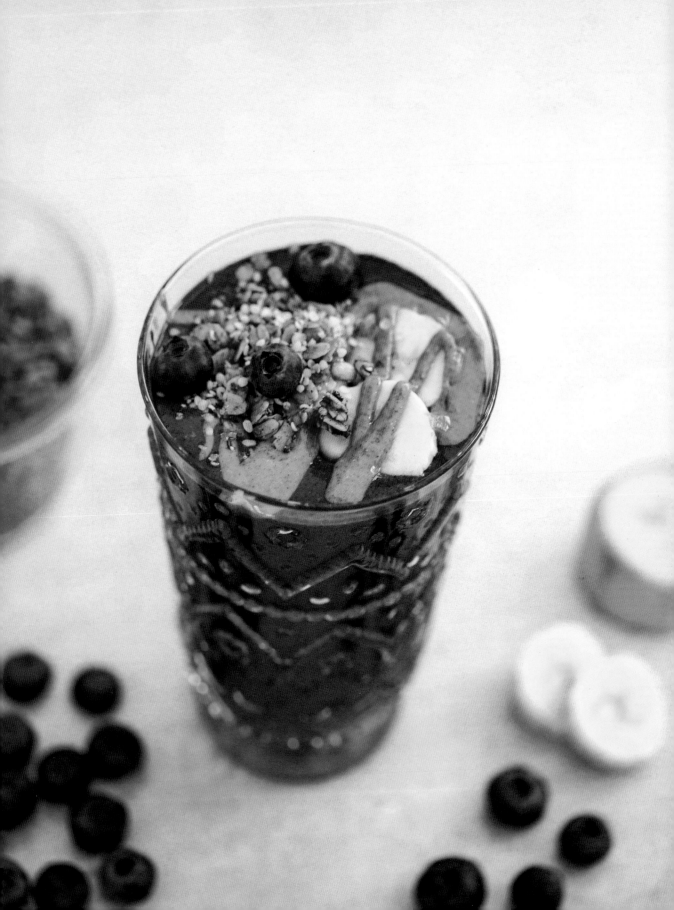

The Ultimate Period Smoothie

Here's your go-to power smoothie for when you have your period, full of all the fruits and greens that are ideal for this phase. Because menstruation weakens your immune system, it's a good time to amp up smoothies with turmeric, ginger, spirulina, and hemp seeds. Hemp seeds are one of my favorite things and are so underrated! They offer lots of protein, healthy omegas, iron, magnesium, and zinc, all of which you need during this time. This smoothie will leave you feeling hydrated, balanced, and truly nourished.

Combine all the ingredients, including any optional add-ins, in a blender. Blend until smooth and creamy. Pour into a cup and sprinkle with your favorite toppings. Serve immediately.

SERVES: 1

1 ½ cups kale, torn (about 2 leaves, de-stemmed)

¾ cup frozen wild blueberries

1 frozen banana

½-inch knob fresh ginger, peeled (or 1 tablespoon ground)

½-inch knob fresh turmeric, peeled (or 1 teaspoon ground)

3 tablespoons hemp seeds

2 tablespoons raw cacao powder

1 tablespoon ground flaxseed

½ teaspoon spirulina powder

1 ½ cups coconut water (or filtered water or nut milk)

Optional add-ins: ½ raw peeled red beet, scoop of plant protein for an extra boost

Optional toppings: extra wild blueberries, drizzle of nut butter, granola

Winter Wild Blueberry Super "Cereal"

SERVES: 1

1 ½ cups coconut milk

¾ cup frozen wild blueberries

2 tablespoons hemp seeds

2 tablespoons shredded coconut

1 tablespoon chia seeds

1 tablespoon ground flaxseed

1 tablespoon cacao nibs

2 dropperfuls liquid stevia (or 1 tablespoon pure maple syrup)

Optional add-ins: sliced banana, spoonful of almond butter

Optional toppings: granola, ground cinnamon, extra hemp seeds, and shredded coconut

This fun play on cold "cereal" is perfect for mornings when you don't have much time or energy. A lightly sweet and deliciously filling bowl, it's loaded with healthy fats, protein, and fiber. The wild blueberries steal the show and turn the coconut milk into a beautiful hue of blue. Did you know wild blueberries have twice the antioxidant capacity per serving as regular ones? Not all blueberries are created equal! (If you can't find wild blueberries in the store, though, the regular variety will work fine in this recipe.) Sprinkling in lots of fiber-filled seeds like chia, flax, and hemp makes this oh-so-satisfying and a much healthier alternative to your typical store-bought cereal breakfast.

Combine all the ingredients, including any optional add-ins, in a serving bowl and stir. Let sit for a few minutes so the seeds start absorbing the coconut milk and the blueberries start to thaw. Then sprinkle on the optional toppings and serve. Store leftovers, if there are any.

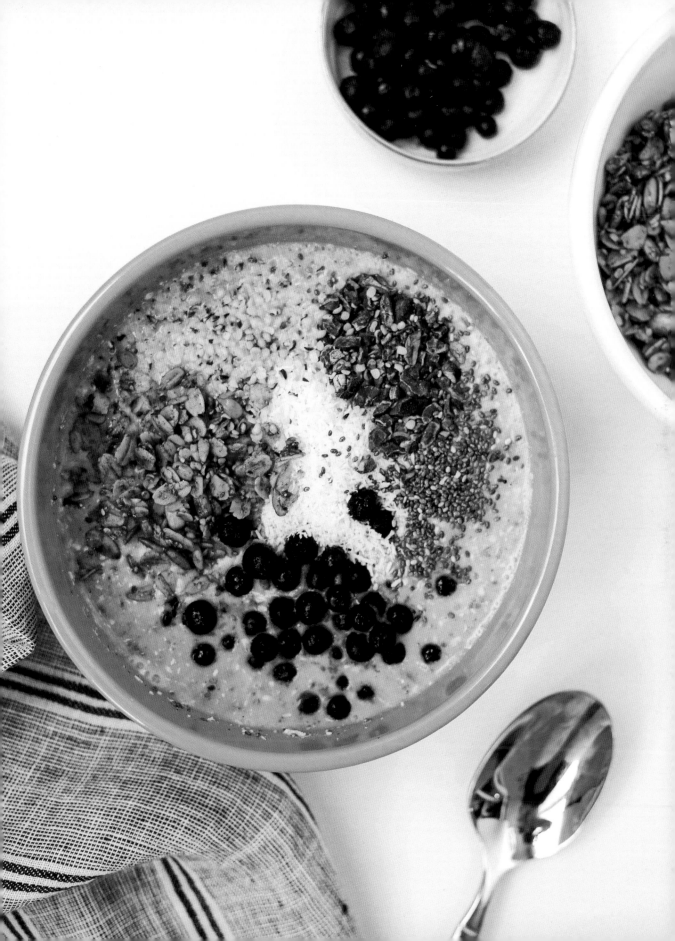

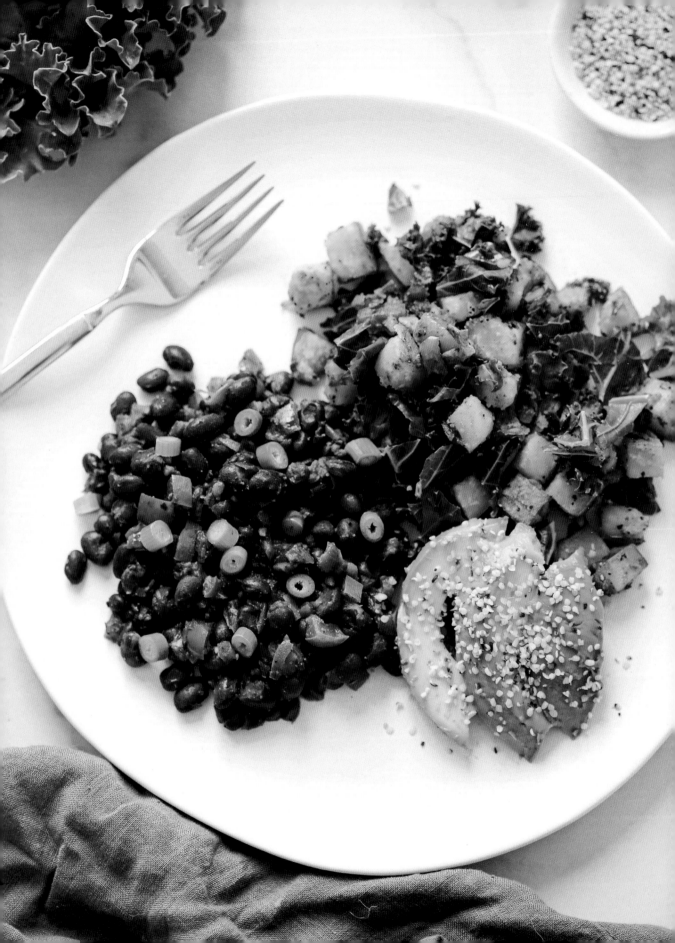

Beans for Breakfast Plate

I know I'm not alone in craving healthy comfort food during my period! This is for a good reason because the body craves foods that keep your uterus warm during this phase. Black beans are one of the best foods to incorporate due to their high protein, fiber, iron, calcium, and potassium content. This helps re-mineralize the body, which is important because we lose a lot of minerals during the menstrual phase. And we can't forget about our greens, which is why I added kale to the mix. Feel free to sprinkle with dulse flakes for extra good measure as they provide high amounts of iodine for thyroid health.

Heat the avocado oil in a medium saucepan over medium-high heat. Add the onion and sauté until it turns translucent and begins to brown, about 5 minutes. Add the bell pepper and garlic and cook for 3 more minutes. Add all the remaining ingredients for the black beans and stir until coated, then reduce the heat, cover, and simmer for 7–8 minutes.

Meanwhile, wash the potatoes, set them on top of a wet paper towel, and microwave for 5 minutes (this will help them cook faster). Remove the potatoes from the microwave and let cool for a few minutes, then carefully cube them into small pieces and set aside.

Heat the remaining oil in a frying pan over medium-high heat. Once hot, add the onion and sauté until it turns translucent and begins to brown, about 5 minutes. Add the bell pepper, sea salt, black pepper, paprika, chili powder, and red pepper flakes, if using, and stir until well coated. Cook for 2–3 minutes, then stir in the potatoes and water. Cover to steam cook for 10 minutes, stirring occasionally. Then tilt the lid to let out some of the steam and cook (partially covered) for 5 more minutes. Reduce the heat to low, stir in the kale, and cook for 2 minutes, or until wilted.

Divide the beans and potatoes between two plates, add any optional toppings, and serve. Store leftovers in an airtight container in the refrigerator for up to 3 days.

SERVES: 2

BLACK BEANS

1 tablespoon avocado oil

¼ red onion, chopped

½ bell pepper (any color), chopped

1 clove garlic, minced

1 (15-ounce) can black beans, drained and rinsed

1 ½ teaspoons ground cumin

1 ½ teaspoons dried oregano

½ teaspoon sea salt

2 tablespoons filtered water

1 teaspoon red wine vinegar

SAUTÉ

2 small red or gold potatoes

1 tablespoon avocado oil

¼ red onion, chopped

½ bell pepper (any color), chopped

½ teaspoon sea salt

½ teaspoon black pepper

½ teaspoon paprika

½ teaspoon chili powder

¼ teaspoon red pepper flakes (optional)

¼ cup filtered water

1 ½ cups kale, chopped (about 2 leaves, de-stemmed)

Optional toppings: avocado slices, dulse flakes

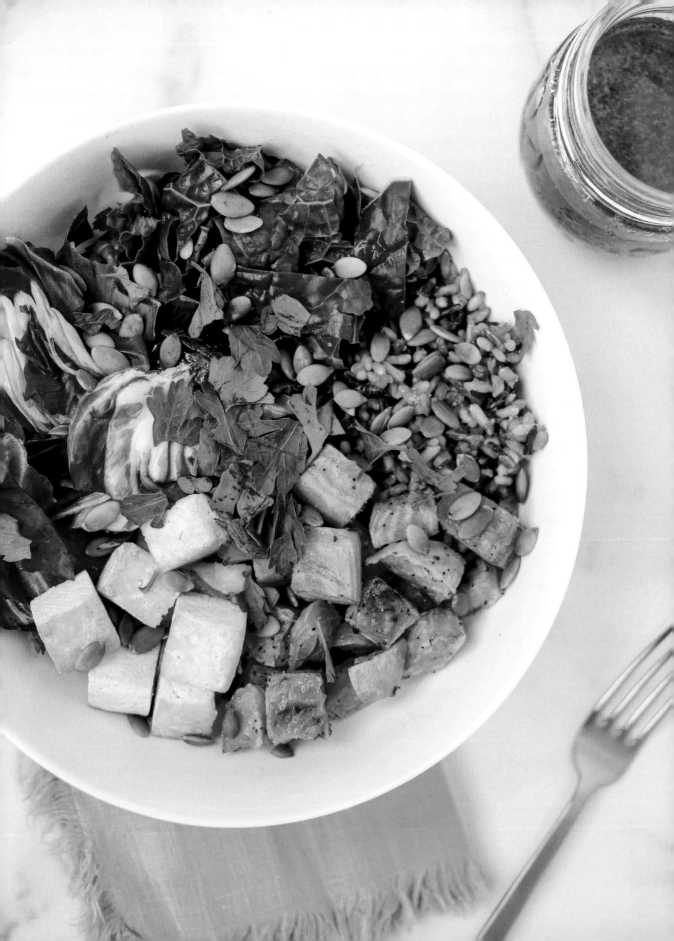

Prep Time: 15 minutes   **Cook Time:** 60 minutes   **Total Time:** 75 minutes

Wild Rice Goldie Glow Bowl

If I'm feeling anxious—which can happen during my period—I focus on grounding foods like beets. They are a superfood with their high fiber, iron, magnesium, vitamin C, and vitamin B6 content. Paired with comforting wild rice and crispy tofu, the beets in this earthy and salty glow bowl will brighten your day and bring you back to earth. You can also quickly prep this lunch ahead of time to grab on busy days!

Preheat the oven to 400°F. Cut the green leafy tops off the beets and save the greens for another recipe or use (smoothies, sautés, etc.). Scrub the beets thoroughly, then wrap them loosely in aluminum foil (no need to dry them before wrapping).

Pour 2 tablespoons of water onto a rimmed baking sheet and place the wrapped beets on the sheet. Roast on the middle rack of your oven for 50–60 minutes.

Meanwhile, combine the wild rice and water in a medium saucepan over high heat. Bring to a boil, then cover and reduce the heat to simmer for 45 minutes. When the rice is done, turn off the heat and keep the lid on until ready to serve.

Check the beets after about 50 minutes. They are done when a fork can easily pierce through to the center of the beet. Small beets will cook more quickly. Set the beets aside to cool for a few minutes. Once they are cool enough to handle, hold one of the beets in a paper towel and use the edges of the paper towel to rub the skin away. It should peel away easily. If not, the beets likely need to cook a little longer. When all the beets are ready, peel, chop, and set aside.

SERVES: 2

RICE BOWL

2 medium-sized raw golden beets

½ cup dry wild rice

1 ¼ cups filtered water

1 tablespoon avocado oil

½ block extra-firm tofu, drained and cubed (see note)

1 bunch lacinato kale, de-stemmed and chopped

½ head radicchio, sliced (optional)

Optional toppings: pepitas, dulse flakes, avocado

SIMPLE ONE-MINUTE DRESSING

¼ cup olive oil

¼ cup apple cider vinegar

1 tablespoon pure maple syrup

1 teaspoon Dijon mustard

Pinch of sea salt and black pepper

recipe continues

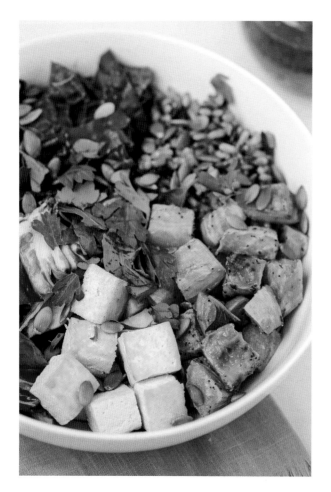

Heat the avocado oil in a frying pan over medium heat. Once hot, add the tofu and fry for 4–5 minutes on each side, until golden brown. Once all sides are browned, reduce the heat, stir in the kale, and cook for 2 minutes, until wilted and warmed.

Whisk all the ingredients for the dressing together in a small bowl, or combine in a blender for a creamier consistency.

To assemble, divide the wild rice between two bowls and top with the golden beets, tofu, kale, and radicchio, if using. Drizzle with the simple dressing, top with any optional toppings, and serve warm. Store leftovers in an airtight container in the refrigerator for up to 3 days.

Note: It's not necessary to press the tofu for this recipe, but you could if you have the extra time; just use a tofu press for 10 minutes, until most of the water is pressed out, or do it yourself with tools you already have in your home. Follow the instructions on page 56.

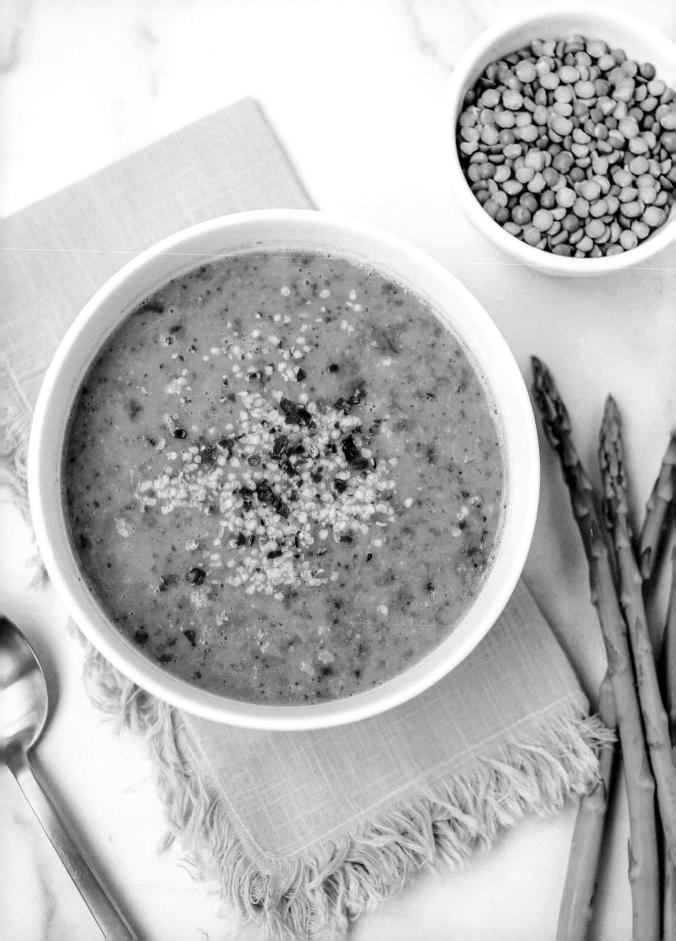

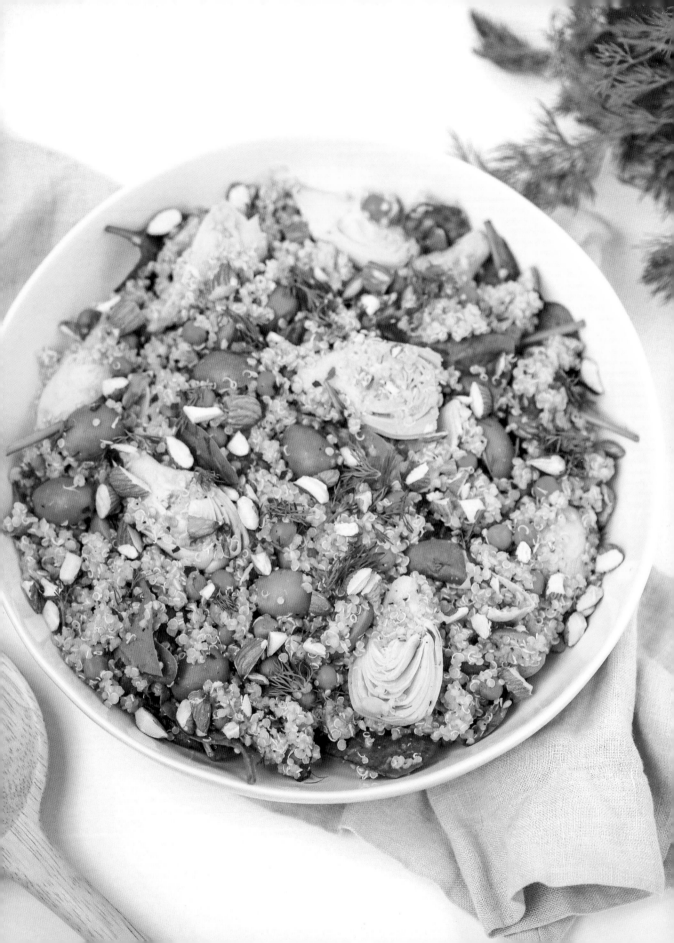

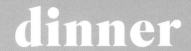

Prep Time: 15 minutes   Cook Time: 15 minutes   Total Time: 30 minutes

Spring Lemon and Dill Artichoke Quinoa

This vibrant dinner is full of spring vibes and the freshest of fresh ingredients. The acidic tang of the artichokes and salt of the green olives, paired with the smooth lemon-dill sauce and crunchy almonds, will have you reaching for seconds. Artichokes have a wonderful velvety texture and are high in vitamin C and magnesium. Olives provide healthy fats, and quinoa is a solid source of protein. I like to toss in some fresh spinach for extra greens.

Combine the quinoa and water in a medium saucepan over medium-high heat. Bring to a boil. Reduce the heat to low, cover, and simmer for 15 minutes, or until all the water is absorbed.

Combine all the ingredients for the sauce in a blender and blend until smooth. Set aside.

Combine the spinach, artichokes, green peas, green olives, and crushed almonds in a large salad bowl. Pour the cooked quinoa over the top, along with the Lemon-Dill Sauce. Toss well to combine. Serve immediately, or transfer to an airtight container and store in the refrigerator for up to 3 days.

SERVES: 3–4

QUINOA MIXTURE

1 cup quinoa

2 cups filtered water

2 cups fresh baby spinach

1 (14-ounce) can artichokes, drained

1 cup green peas (thawed if frozen)

½ cup green olives, halved

2 tablespoons crushed almonds

LEMON-DILL SAUCE

½ cup light coconut milk

Zest and juice of 1 lemon

½ cup fresh dill

1 clove garlic

1 teaspoon sea salt

1 teaspoon black pepper

¼ teaspoon onion powder

½ teaspoon red pepper flakes (optional)

Sticky Tofu Teriyaki

SERVES: 2–3

TOFU

1 (14-ounce) package extra-firm tofu

1 tablespoon coconut oil, divided

2–3 green onions, chopped

1-inch knob fresh ginger, peeled and minced (or 1 tablespoon ground)

1 clove garlic, minced

1 bell pepper, sliced thin

2 large carrots, sliced

2 cups broccoli florets

¼ cup fresh basil, chopped (optional)

Cooked brown or jasmine rice (optional, for serving)

Optional toppings: crushed almonds, cilantro, extra basil, fresh lime juice, red pepper flakes

For anyone who thinks tofu is boring, this dish is here to prove you wrong. It's all about how you flavor and cook the tofu! Plus, the sauce really does get sticky—it's the magic touch. Not to mention, tofu provides an adequate amount of vitamin B6, an essential vitamin for detoxification and healthy ovulation. We use lots of fiber-rich broccoli, carrots, and bell pepper, making for a filling and balanced dinner. I love the flavor combo here of salty, sour, and slightly sweet. Yum! One thing to note: It's important to buy organic tofu as non-organic can contain genetically modified soybeans.

Optional: Pressing tofu isn't a must, but doing so helps remove the excess water and makes the cooked tofu crispier. To press your tofu, you can drain it and use a store-bought tofu press, or you can do it yourself. Cut the block crosswise into 1-inch strips. Lay two paper towels or one clean kitchen towel on a baking sheet and place the tofu strips in a single layer on the towels. Lay two more paper towels or another clean kitchen towel on top of the tofu. Place another baking sheet (or any heavy, flat-bottomed object) on top, and add a fairly heavy book on top of that. Set aside for 20–30 minutes.

Cut the tofu into cubes and set aside.

Combine all the ingredients for the sauce (see ingredients to the right) in a small bowl and whisk together until smooth. Set aside.

Heat 1 ½ teaspoons of the coconut oil in a frying pan over medium heat. Once hot, stir in the green onions. Cook for 2–3 minutes, then stir in the ginger and garlic. Cook for 2–3 minutes, stirring occasionally and being careful not to burn. Stir in the bell peppers, carrots, broccoli, and basil, if using. Cover and steam cook for 7–8 minutes, or until the veggies are cooked through. Transfer the veggies to a bowl and set aside.

Heat the remaining 1 ½ teaspoons of coconut oil in the same frying pan over medium-high heat. Once hot, stir in the tofu and fry for about 4 minutes on each side, until golden brown.

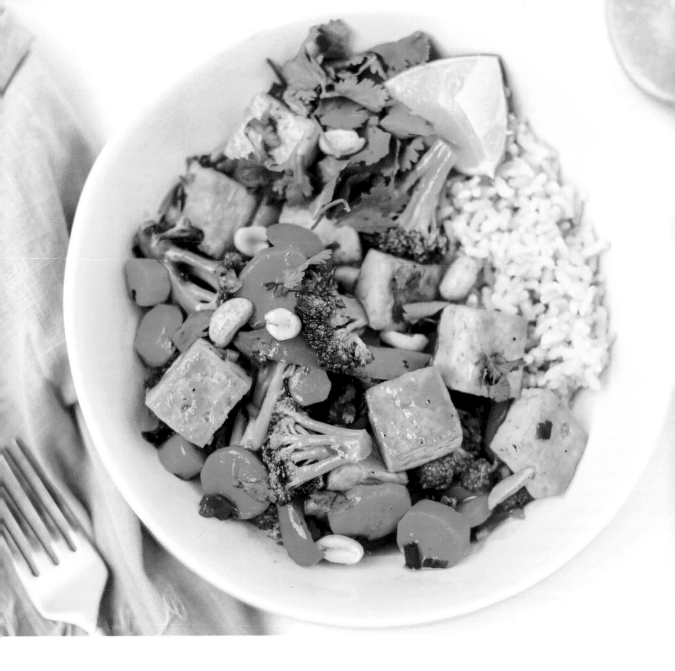

Pour in the Sticky Sauce while stirring constantly (I like to use a spatula for this) and watch it transform and get sticky over the span of a few minutes. Lower the heat, then add the cooked vegetables and stir until well combined and coated with the sticky sauce.

Divide the tofu among plates, top with any optional toppings, and serve alone or alongside rice. Store leftovers in an airtight container in the refrigerator for up to 3 days.

STICKY SAUCE

¼ cup filtered water

3 tablespoons tamari

2 tablespoons rice vinegar

1 ½ tablespoons pure maple syrup

1 tablespoon tapioca starch

1 tablespoon sriracha (or chili sauce, optional)

Nutty Green Bean Zoodle Sauté

SERVES: 2

ZOODLE SAUTÉ

1 tablespoon avocado oil
(or coconut oil)

1 shallot, diced

1 clove garlic, minced

Pinch of sea salt and black pepper

Pinch of red pepper flakes (optional)

2 cups fresh green beans, trimmed
(I do not recommend frozen)

2 medium-sized zucchini, spiralized

Juice of ½ lemon

BRAZIL NUT CRUMBLE

¼ cup Brazil nuts

¼ cup nutritional yeast

2 tablespoons hemp seeds

Basic, bright, and lemony, this recipe is just right for the spring phase. Because you want to optimize digestion at this time, it's important to keep your meals as simple and whole as possible. Real, whole-food ingredients are much easier on the body's digestion. I love zucchini noodles (also known as "zoodles") for the follicular phase because they're light and filled with vitamin C and vitamin B6, which are important vitamins for liver detoxification. I chose Brazil nuts because they're high in selenium, a crucial mineral for healthy ovarian follicle development, and bring a satisfying crunch to this dish.

Heat the avocado oil in a large skillet over medium heat. Once hot, add the shallot and sauté for 3–4 minutes. Stir in the garlic, sea salt, black pepper, and red pepper flakes, if using, and cook, stirring occasionally for 2–3 more minutes, until fragrant. Stir in the green beans and cover to steam cook for 7–8 minutes.

Meanwhile, combine all the ingredients for the Brazil Nut Crumble in a food processor and pulse until crumbly, like breadcrumbs.

Stir the zucchini, lemon juice, and Brazil Nut Crumble into the green bean mixture and cover to slightly cook the zucchini noodles for 3 minutes. Taste test and add more sea salt if needed, then turn off the heat.

Divide between two bowls and serve immediately. Store leftovers in the refrigerator for up to 3 days.

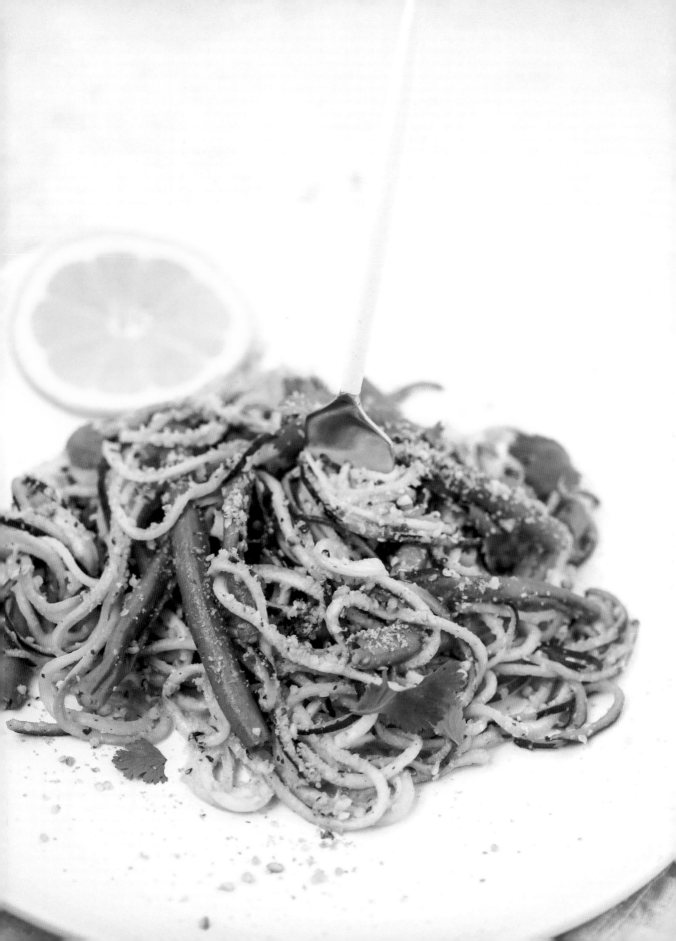

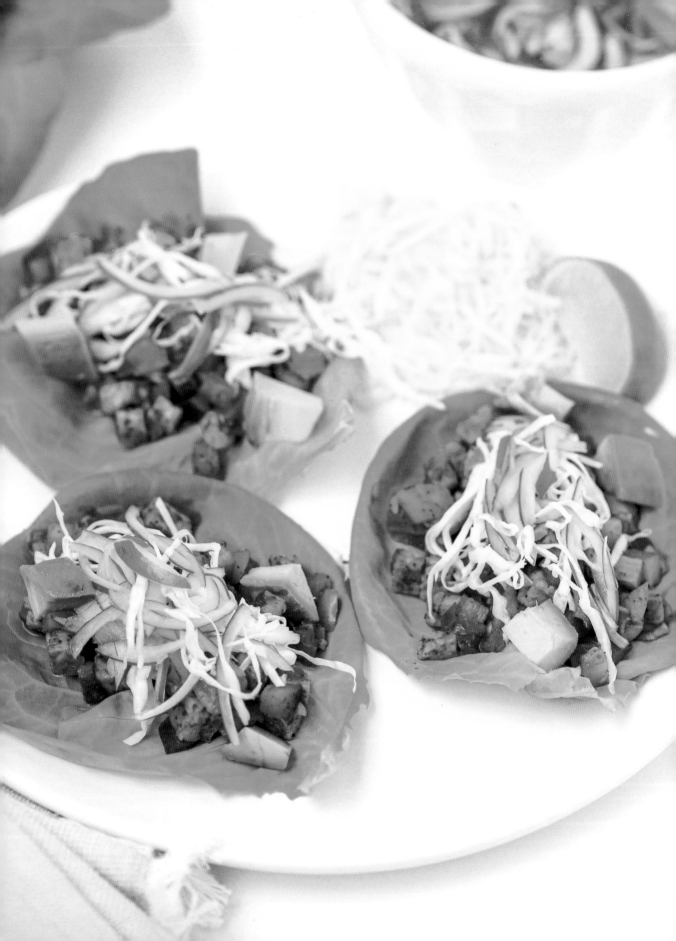

Tempeh Taco Lettuce Wraps with Quick-Pickled Red Onions

At this time in my cycle, I rarely want a heavy meal. We tend to have more energy during the follicular phase, and lighter meals make you feel good while not weighing you down! That doesn't mean we skimp on nutrition, though. During this phase, I like to use tempeh instead of beans or legumes because it's easier to digest. These tacos make me feel amazing—I could eat them every day. The soft butter lettuce leaves hold up well, and the quick-pickled red onions are delectably tangy and tie all the flavors together!

To pickle the red onion, place it in a small bowl. Combine the apple cider vinegar, sea salt, and coconut sugar and pour the mixture over the onions. Push them down with a spoon to submerge. Let sit at room temperature for at least 20 minutes while you prepare the lettuce wraps. If making ahead, store in the refrigerator after 20 minutes.

Meanwhile, heat the avocado oil in a large skillet over medium heat. Once hot, add the onion and sauté for 3–4 minutes or until translucent. Stir in the bell pepper, zucchini, sea salt, and black pepper and cook, stirring occasionally for 3–4 minutes. Stir in the tempeh, chili powder, cumin, paprika, and water. Cover and let simmer for 15–20 minutes.

Serve the tempeh mixture with the green cabbage, lettuce leaves, quick-pickled red onions, and optional toppings on the side, and let your guests assemble their own wraps. Store leftovers in an airtight container in the refrigerator for up to 3 days.

SERVES: 3

TACO LETTUCE WRAPS

1 tablespoon avocado oil

¼ red onion, chopped

1 bell pepper, chopped small

1 large zucchini, chopped small

¾ teaspoon sea salt

¾ teaspoon black pepper

1 (8-ounce) package tempeh, chopped small

2 teaspoons chili powder

2 teaspoons ground cumin

2 teaspoons paprika

½ cup filtered water

1 cup shredded green cabbage

9 butter lettuce leaves

Optional toppings: avocado, pico de gallo, fresh lime, pickled onions

QUICK-PICKLED RED ONIONS

1 cup very thinly sliced red onion (I use a mandoline slicer)

½ cup apple cider vinegar

½ teaspoon sea salt

½ teaspoon coconut sugar

Macadamia Turmeric Coconut Curry

SERVES: 4–5

1 cup yellow lentils

3 ½ cups filtered water, divided

1 tablespoon avocado oil

1 shallot, chopped

2–3 tablespoons red curry paste (to taste)

2 cloves garlic, minced

1 tablespoon minced fresh ginger

½ teaspoon sea salt

½ teaspoon black pepper

¼ teaspoon red pepper flakes (optional)

2 large carrots, chopped

6 ounces (or 3/4 cup) sugar snap peas

2 cups broccoli florets

1 (13.5-ounce) can light coconut milk

1 tablespoon pure maple syrup

1 teaspoon ground turmeric

Juice of 1 lime (about 2 tablespoons)

¼ cup macadamia nuts, for topping

Cooked jasmine rice (optional, for serving)

Optional toppings: cilantro, extra fresh lime juice, red pepper flakes

This comforting coconut curry is beautifully golden and full of anti-inflammatory properties. I chose yellow lentils for their protein, fiber, and easy digestibility. The golden sauce is not too rich or overpowering, which is the case with some curries. The dish is perfectly balanced and grounding, and it's even more satisfying when paired with jasmine rice.

Soak the lentils in enough water to cover for 15 minutes. Drain and rinse the lentils, then combine them with 3 cups of the water in a pot on the stove. Bring to a boil, then reduce the heat to simmer, uncovered, for 20 minutes or until most of the water is absorbed. Drain any remaining water. Set aside.

Meanwhile, heat the avocado oil in a large pot or Dutch oven over medium-high heat. Once hot, add the shallot and sauté for 3–4 minutes. Stir in the red curry paste, garlic, ginger, sea salt, black pepper, and red pepper flakes, if using. Cook for 2–3 minutes, stirring occasionally, then stir in the carrots, sugar snap peas, and broccoli. Cover to steam cook for 5 minutes.

Pour in the cooked lentils, the remaining ½ cup water, and the coconut milk, maple syrup, and turmeric. Bring to a slight boil, then cover and reduce the heat to simmer for 10–15 minutes or until the veggies are cooked through. Turn off the heat and stir in the lime juice.

Divide the curry among bowls alongside the jasmine rice, if using, and top each serving with macadamia nuts and any other additional toppings. Store leftovers in an airtight container in the refrigerator for up to 3 days, or in the freezer for up to 3 months.

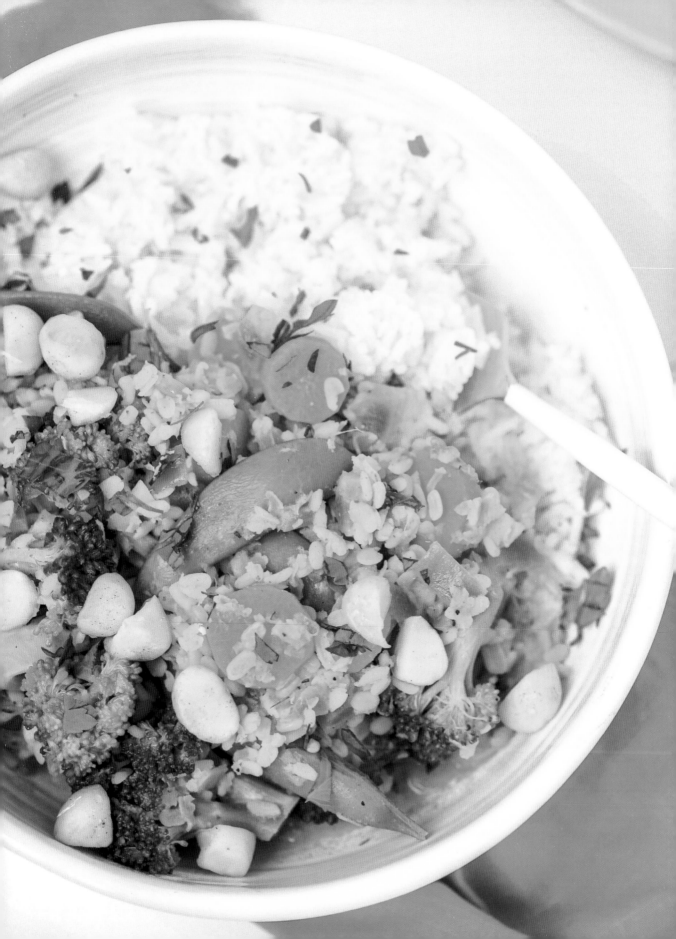

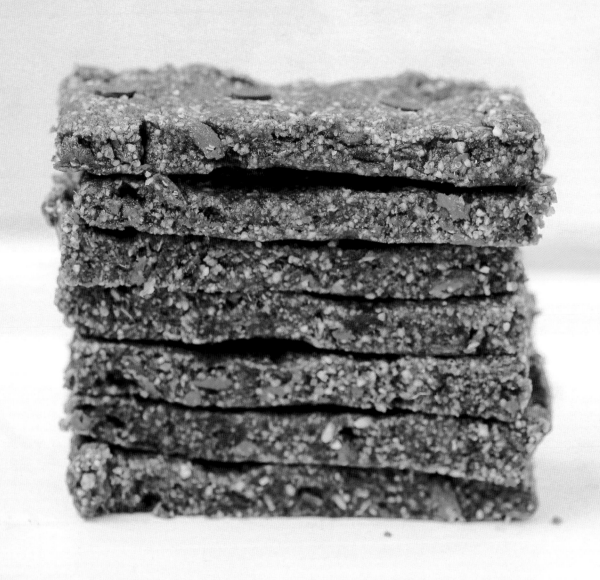

Prep Time: 50 minutes   **Total Time:** 50 minutes

Happy Hormone Superfood Snack Bars

These bars are so yummy—they taste like an upgraded Lärabar or gooey granola bar. Plus, they're super easy to make and keep well so that you can grab them for a satisfying snack on the go. All you need is a food processor and square baking dish! They are filled with fiber, protein, and antioxidants, and have the appropriate seeds for seed cycling during your follicular phase. I like to prep these on Sundays for the week ahead.

MAKES: 8 BARS

1 cup pitted medjool dates (10–12 dates)

½ cup goji berries

¾ cup almonds

½ cup pepitas

3 tablespoons hemp seeds

2 tablespoons ground flaxseed

2 ½ teaspoons ground cinnamon

¼ teaspoon sea salt

Optional topping: vegan chocolate chips

Soak the medjool dates and goji berries in hot water for 10 minutes, to soften. Drain and set aside.

Combine the almonds and pepitas in a food processor and blend into a crumbly flour. No worries if there are some bigger chunks.

Add the hemp seeds, ground flaxseed, cinnamon, and sea salt and blend until well combined. Add the soaked dates and goji berries and pulse/blend until it forms a sticky, thick dough.

Line an 8x8-inch square baking pan with parchment paper, leaving some overhang on each side. Transfer the dough to the pan and press it into the pan with your hands. It helps if your hands are wet, because the dough is very sticky. You can also use a flat-bottomed measuring cup to flatten out the dough.

Refrigerate for 20–30 minutes to set.

Use the edges of the parchment paper to lift the bars out of the pan and onto a cutting board, then slice into 8 bars. Transfer to an airtight container and store in the refrigerator for up to 2 weeks.

Easy Pickled Veggies

SERVES: 6

1 ½ cups fresh trimmed green beans

1 ½ cups sliced carrots

½ shallot, sliced

1–2 cloves garlic, sliced or minced

2–3 sprigs fresh dill

1 cup filtered water

¾ cup white vinegar

1 teaspoon sea salt

¼ teaspoon ground cayenne pepper

These crunchy, spicy, and tangy pickled veggies are the perfect snack. They're also excellent on top of salads. The pickling process is much easier than you think. Once you get the hang of it, you'll be pickling all the time! You just blanch the veggies and bring the brine to a boil, then pour the brine over the veggies in a jar and wait 24 hours. You can also add in your favorite high-flavor veggies like jalapeños, onions, or extra garlic. It's fun to play around with the flavors and find the mix you like best. Not to mention, fermented foods contain live bacteria, which help the breakdown of food during digestion, making these a go-to for the follicular phase.

Fill a large sauté pan with about an inch of water (enough to cover the green beans) and bring to a boil. Add the green beans and carrots, and boil for 2–3 minutes to blanch and slightly soften the veggies. Remove from the heat and transfer the veggies to a large, clean mason jar. Add the shallot, garlic, and dill.

Combine the water, vinegar, sea salt, and cayenne pepper in a medium saucepan to make the brine. Bring to a boil and stir to dissolve the salt. Once the salt is all dissolved, remove from the heat and pour the hot brine into the mason jar. Gently tap the jar against the countertop to remove any air bubbles.

Tightly seal the jar and leave on the countertop for 1 hour to cool to room temperature. Then refrigerate for at least 24 hours before opening the jar. The flavor improves with time! Store the jar in the refrigerator for up to 3–4 weeks.

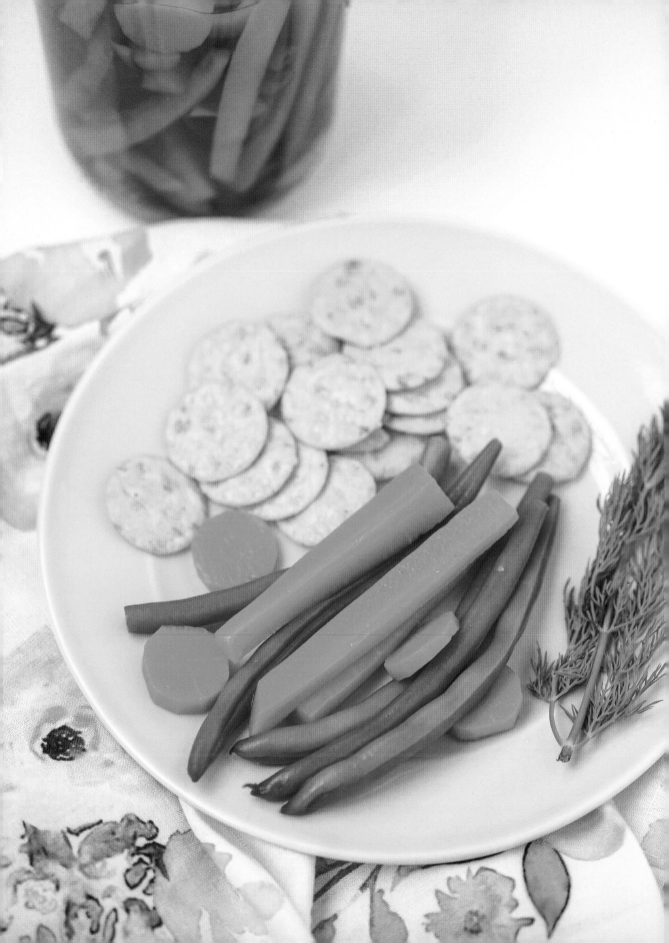

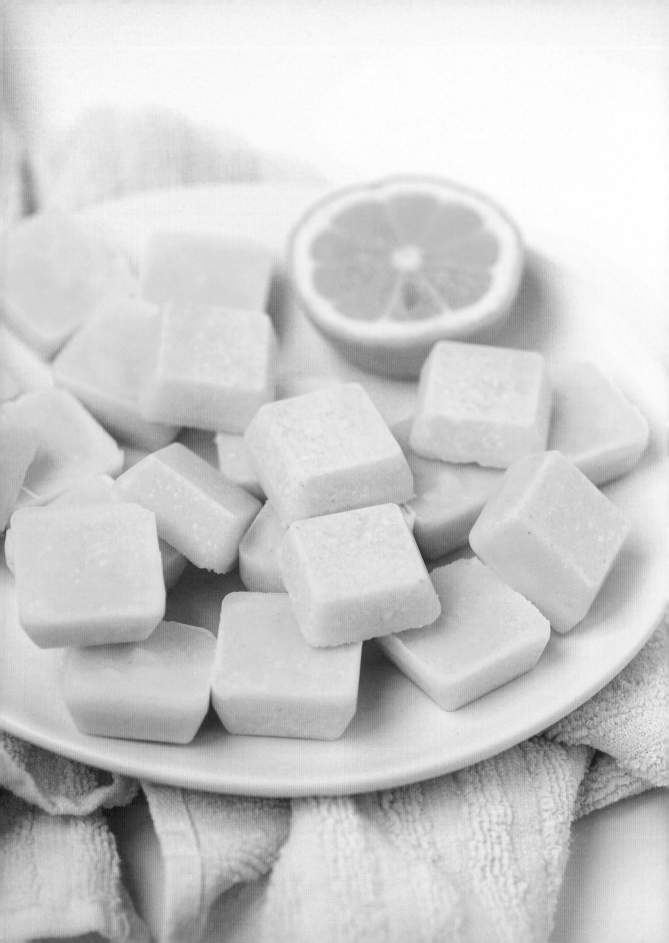

Prep Time: 30 minutes   Freeze Time: 30 minutes   Total Time: 60 minutes

Lemon Fudge Bombs

This one is for my sweet-tooth lemon lovers: silky, smooth, melt-in-your-mouth lemon fudge that is also sugar-free. Yes, please! Super easy and refreshingly tart, these decadent gems make a cooling treat perfect for your follicular phase. I also love their bright and happy neon yellow color! Keep them in the fridge for a sweet fix that won't send you on a sugar spiral.

MAKES: 20 SMALL SQUARES

½ cup coconut butter (or cashew butter, but this will change the color and texture)

½ cup melted coconut oil

2 tablespoons fresh lemon juice

25 drops liquid stevia (or monk fruit drops, or 1 tablespoon pure maple syrup)

5 drops lemon essential oil (optional)

¼ teaspoon ground turmeric

Pinch of sea salt

Line a mini muffin pan with liners, or have a silicone candy mold or ice cube tray ready.

To warm the coconut butter, place the glass jar in a small pot and fill with enough water to come halfway up the sides of the jar. Bring to a boil, then reduce the heat to simmer for 15–20 minutes, or until the coconut butter is stirrable (the consistency will still be very thick).

Combine the warmed coconut butter with all the remaining ingredients in a small mixing bowl and whisk until super smooth and well combined.

Pour about 1 tablespoon of the mixture into each mini muffin liner or mold. Freeze for 30 minutes, then transfer to an airtight container and store in the refrigerator for up to 2 weeks.

Orange Jelly Thumbprint Cookies

MAKES: 12 COOKIES

1 ¼ cups almond flour

¼ cup coconut sugar

½ teaspoon baking soda

½ teaspoon sea salt

¾ cup runny almond butter

1 tablespoon melted coconut oil

1 teaspoon vanilla extract

¼ cup flaxseeds

½ cup natural orange jelly

These grain-free thumbprint cookies are just the cutest. They feel festive and buttery sweet, even though they have no butter at all! You can use any flavor of jelly (as long as it is natural and organic and free of refined sugar); I chose orange since it is good for this phase. Feel free to replace the almond butter with any nut or seed butter you love. Pairing these cookies with tea or decaf coffee has become one of my favorite afternoon treats.

Preheat the oven to 350°F. Line a baking sheet with parchment paper.

Combine the almond flour, coconut sugar, baking soda, and sea salt in a large bowl and whisk together. Add the almond butter, melted coconut oil, and vanilla extract and mix until well combined. If your almond butter is not runny and the dough is a bit crumbly, add water one tablespoon at a time, as needed, until the dough is smooth enough to roll into balls (but not too wet).

Set the flaxseeds in a small bowl. Roll the dough into 1-inch balls, then roll one-half of each ball in the flaxseeds before placing it onto the lined baking sheet. Press the bottom part of a teaspoon into the center of each cookie to form an indent.

Bake the cookies for 10–12 minutes, or until edges are slightly golden brown.

Remove the cookies from the oven. Allow them to cool on the baking sheet for 10 minutes, then fill each cookie with a spoonful of orange jelly.

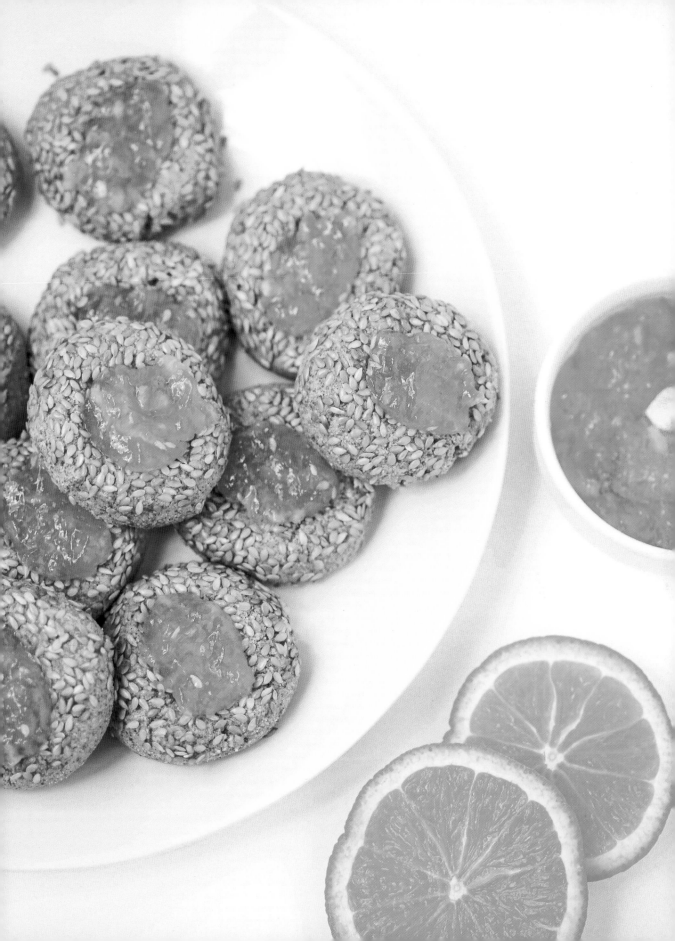

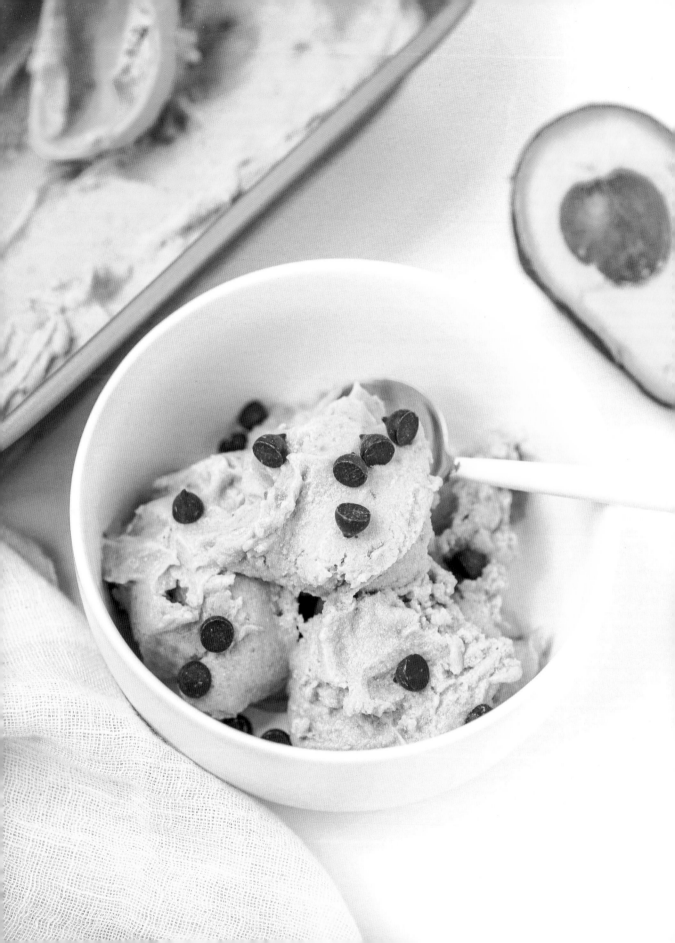

Prep Time: 5 minutes   **Total Time:** 5 minutes

Aloha Detox Smoothie

This liver-detoxifying pink smoothie is a tropical delight! It's an energizing blend made with your digestion in mind. Sometimes we add so many powders and nut butters to our smoothies that they end up sitting in the stomach like a rock, which is really not the point! I kept this one extra light so that it's easy on your digestion first thing in the morning. If you're still hungry, you can have a piece of toast with sunflower seed butter or nut butter afterward. This simple blend is a reminder to be mindful of what we add to our smoothies.

Combine all the ingredients, including any optional add-ins, in a blender. Blend until smooth and creamy. Pour into a glass or jar, sprinkle with any optional toppings, and serve immediately.

SERVES: 1

1 cup frozen strawberries

½ cup frozen pineapple

⅓ cucumber, peeled (you can leave the skin on, but it may affect the color)

½ lemon, peeled

¼ cup fresh cilantro

1-inch knob fresh ginger, peeled

½-inch knob fresh turmeric, peeled

3 tablespoons hemp seeds

½ cup coconut milk

½ cup filtered water

Optional add-ins: dandelion greens, aloe vera, spinach

Optional toppings: shredded coconut, pineapple

Sexy Sunflower Shake

SERVES: 1

1 frozen banana

½ cup frozen cauliflower

2 tablespoons sunflower seed butter (or 2 tablespoons raw sunflower seeds)

2 tablespoons hemp seeds

1 tablespoon chia seeds

1 tablespoon maca powder

1 teaspoon ground cinnamon

1 dropperful liquid stevia

½ cup coconut milk

½ cup filtered water

Optional add-ins: cacao powder, shredded coconut

Optional toppings: hemp seeds, sunflower seeds

This is a thick and sexy morning shake that contains maca, which an adaptogen that not only balances hormones but also boosts libido. It's perfect for the ovulatory phase (unless you're NOT trying to get pregnant). This adaptogen can also help you manage stress levels and keep a balanced mood. The sunflower seed butter provides lots of gut-loving fiber and nourishing nutrients like iron (always important for plant-based eaters) and Vitamin E, a free-radical-fighting antioxidant.

Combine all the ingredients, including any optional add-ins, in a blender. Blend until smooth and creamy. Pour into a glass or jar, sprinkle with any optional toppings, and serve immediately.

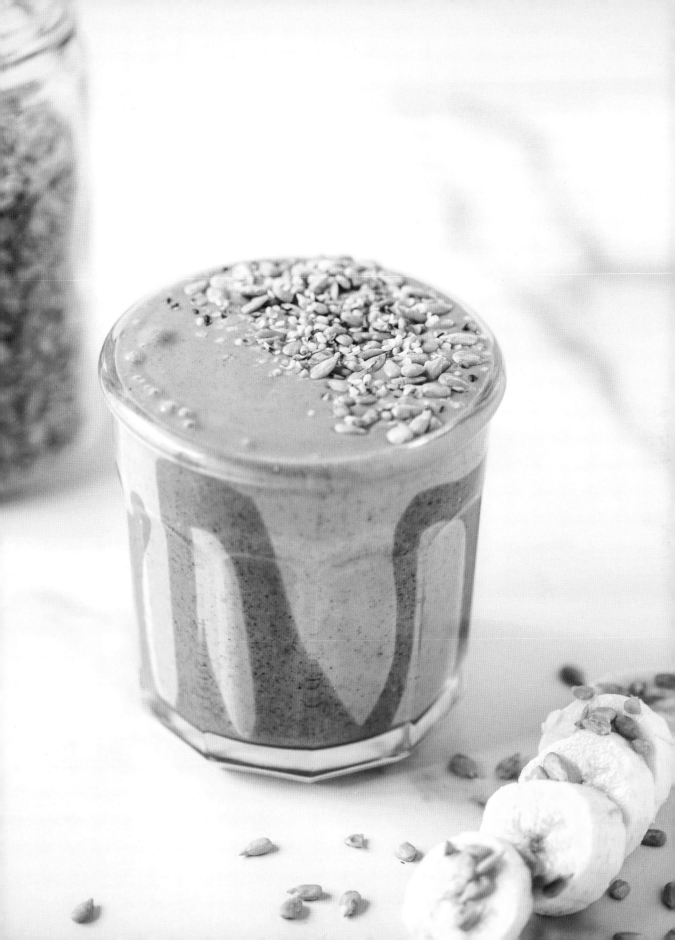

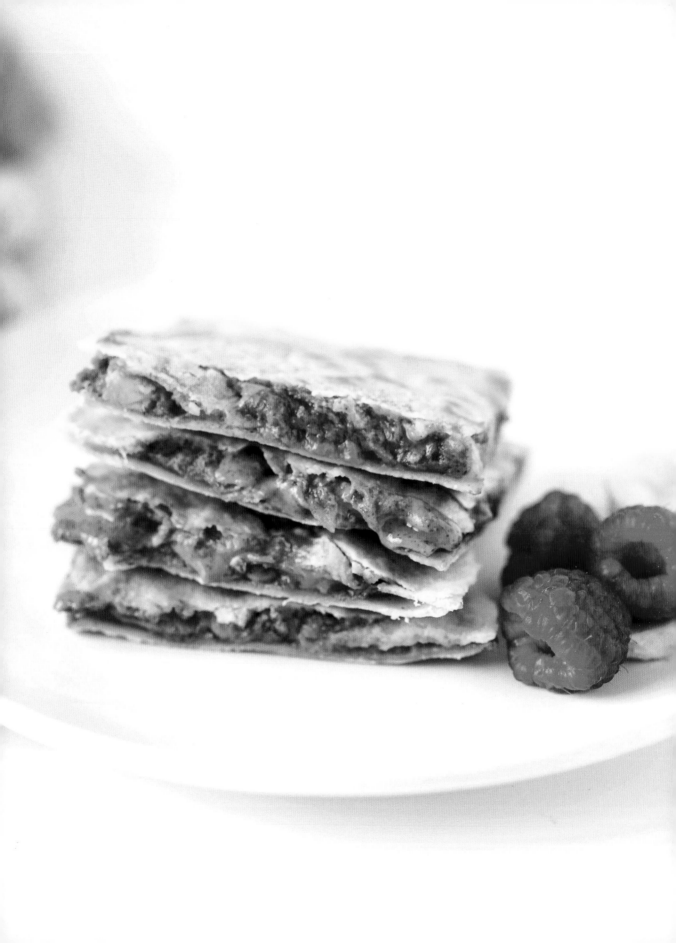

Raspberry–Almond Butter Breakfast Quesadilla

These are such a yummy change of pace from toast, perfect for mornings when you don't have much time and are in the mood for a hint of something sweet. Juicy raspberries paired with creamy bananas and silky almond butter make for a heavenly combo. Feel free to add a vegan protein shake on the side (such as the Sexy Sunflower Shake on page 116) if you need a little more protein to get your day started.

SERVES: 1

2 10-inch gluten-free tortillas of choice (I use Siete almond flour tortillas)

2 tablespoons almond butter

½ ripe banana, sliced

¼ cup raspberries

Sprinkle of ground cinnamon (optional)

Heat a skillet over medium heat. Spray the pan with nonstick cooking spray.

Spread 1 tablespoon of almond butter evenly on each tortilla. Place the banana slices and raspberries on one tortilla. Mash the raspberries down with a fork to make them flatter. Sprinkle with a little cinnamon, if using, and top with the remaining tortilla, almond butter side down.

When the skillet is hot, add the quesadilla. Press down on it gently to help the quesadilla stick together. After 2–3 minutes (or when golden brown), flip the quesadilla. Cut into quarters and serve. Best when eaten immediately.

Papaya Tahini Fruit Boat

SERVES: 1

½ ripe red papaya, seeds removed

½ banana, sliced

½ kiwi, chopped

2 strawberries, chopped

1 tablespoon tahini

1 tablespoon shredded coconut

1 teaspoon chia seeds

1 teaspoon hemp seeds

My dream breakfast. Fresh and juicy red papaya with bites of tropical fruit, shredded coconut, and drizzles of creamy tahini. It is heaven on earth. Ovulation is best supported with lots of raw fruits and veggies, hence this beautiful fruit boat. Fruit should not be feared, especially papaya, because when ripe, it's sweet and luscious. I'm trying to get you to branch out and not buy the same fruits week after week, but instead to expand your horizons and feed your microbes with a different variety of fruit and fiber. I like to buy unripe papayas that are a mixture of green and yellow, with little to no blemishes. You'll know they are ripe when they turn bright yellow and are soft enough that you can almost puncture through the skin with your finger. To eat it, just slice the fruit in half and scoop out the seeds with a spoon. Papaya is an amazing source of fiber, vitamin C, vitamin A, and the digestive enzyme called papain.

Fill the middle of the papaya with the banana, kiwi, and strawberries. Drizzle with the tahini and sprinkle with the coconut, chia seeds, and hemp seeds. Serve immediately and eat with a big spoon! Store the remaining half of the papaya in a container or wrapped in plastic in the refrigerator for up to 2 days.

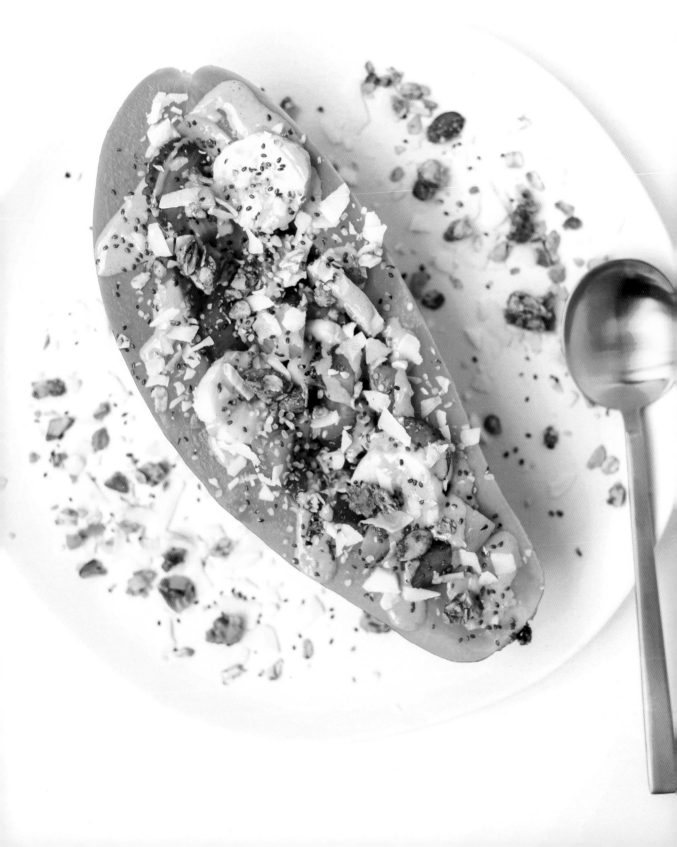

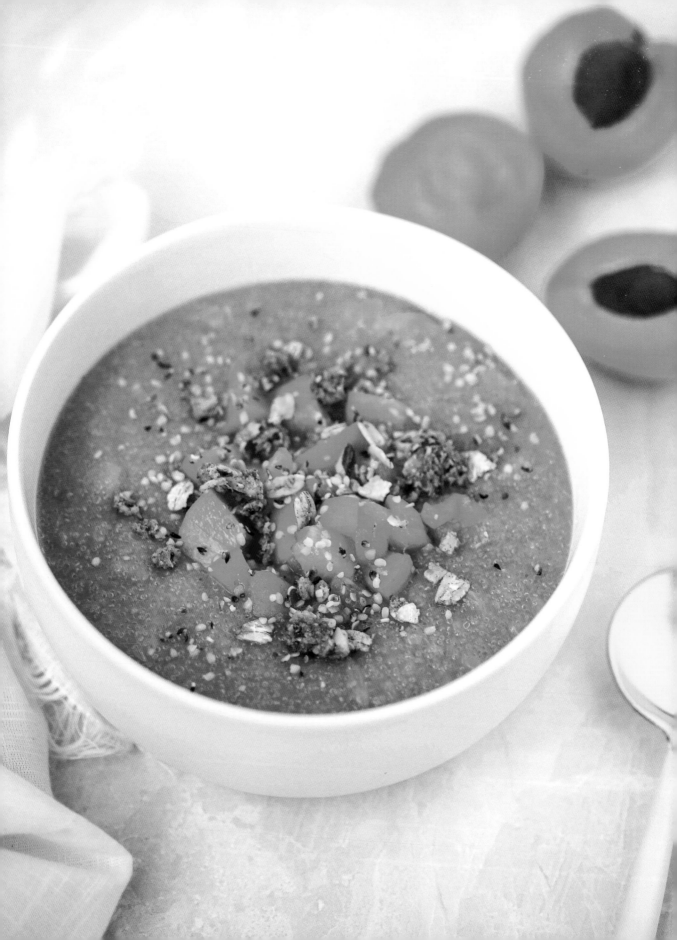

Apricot Amaranth Porridge

There are lots of fun grains to try for breakfast besides oats or quinoa! Amaranth is one of my favorites because it is a complete protein and contains lysine, an amino acid that most grains lack. It's best to choose gluten-free grains when balancing hormones because gluten can be inflammatory for a lot of people. When cooked, amaranth has a sticky consistency, making it perfect for porridge or polenta. The apricots bring a sweet flavor while adding lots of fiber, vitamin A, and vitamin C!

It's really important to rinse off the amaranth first! I do this using a nut milk bag because the amaranth grain is so teeny.

Combine the amaranth, coconut milk, water, maple syrup, vanilla extract, cinnamon, and sea salt in a small saucepan and whisk until smooth. Bring to a boil, then reduce the heat to simmer. Add the diced apricots and cover to simmer for 25 minutes, stirring occasionally, until all the water is absorbed. Spoon into a bowl, sprinkle with any optional toppings, and serve. Store leftovers in an airtight container in the refrigerator for up to 2 days.

SERVES: 2

½ cup amaranth, rinsed

1 cup coconut milk

½ cup filtered water

1 tablespoon pure maple syrup

½ teaspoon vanilla extract

½ teaspoon ground cinnamon

Pinch of sea salt

3 apricots, diced

Optional toppings: hemp seeds, granola, extra coconut milk, extra drizzle of maple syrup

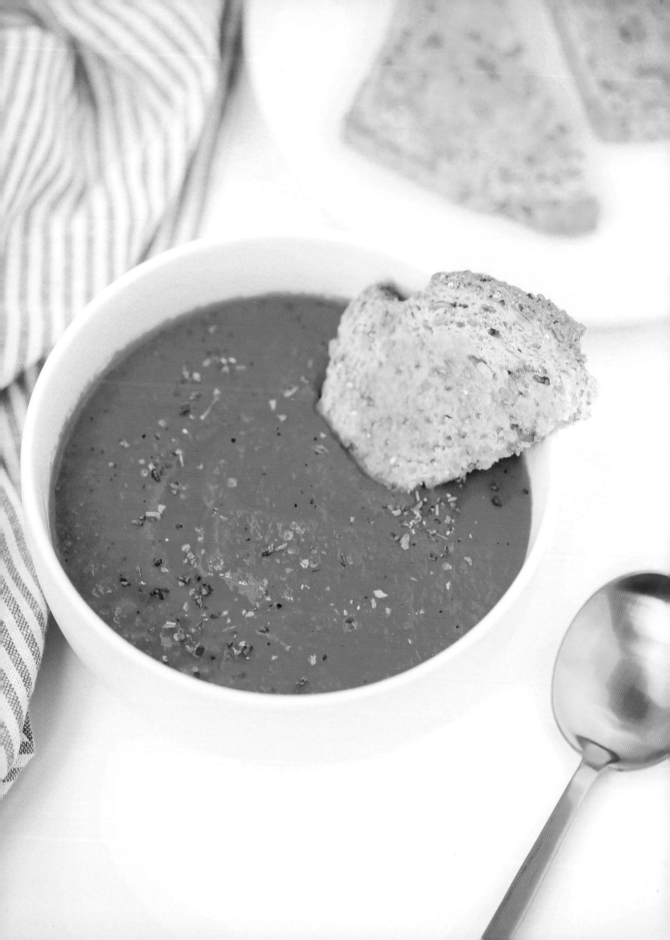

Prep Time: 10 minutes   **Cook Time:** 30 minutes   **Total Time:** 40 minutes

Tomato and Roasted Red Pepper Coconut Soup

This lusciously comforting tomato soup is served up best with toasted gluten-free bread. This one comes together quickly and is great for meal prepping. It has a light summer vibe to it, but it is perfect when you're craving something warm (rather than raw) while you're ovulating. Even though it is dairy free, the coconut gives this soup a pleasant creaminess. The flavor is bright and tangy. Tomatoes are high in vitamin A and vitamin C, and the red bell peppers are a great source of vitamin C as well!

SERVES: 4–5

1 tablespoon coconut oil

½ yellow onion, diced

3 medium carrots, chopped

1 clove garlic, minced

1 (28-ounce) can crushed tomatoes (not drained)

1 (12-ounce) jar roasted red peppers, drained and rinsed

7 ounces light canned coconut milk (half a 13.5-ounce can)

1 teaspoon pure maple syrup

1 ½ teaspoons Italian herb seasoning

1 teaspoon ground turmeric

1 teaspoon sea salt

½ teaspoon black pepper

Juice of ½ lemon

Crusty bread (optional, for serving)

Heat the coconut oil in a large pot over medium heat. Add the onion and sauté for 3–4 minutes. Stir in the carrots and garlic and sauté for 2–3 minutes more. Pour in the crushed tomatoes, roasted red peppers, coconut milk, maple syrup, Italian herb seasoning, turmeric, sea salt, and black pepper. Bring to a boil, then reduce the heat to simmer for 20 minutes. Turn off the heat and stir in the lemon juice.

Using a hand immersion blender, carefully blend the soup until you reach the desired consistency. I prefer it really smooth and creamy. You can also transfer the soup to a high-speed blender, working in batches if necessary, and blend until smooth. Be very careful since the soup is hot! Stop blending once in a while to let out the hot air and prevent a soup explosion!

To serve, divide the soup among bowls. This soup is great when paired with crusty bread spread with some vegan butter or coconut oil on the side. Store leftovers in an airtight container in the refrigerator for up to 4 days, or store in the freezer for up to 2 months.

Jicama Corn Tacos

SERVES: 1–2

5 ounces jicama, cut into sticks
(I like to buy these presliced from
Trader Joe's)

Juice of ½ lime

1 teaspoon chili powder

½ teaspoon sea salt

Dash of ground cayenne pepper
(optional)

3–4 corn tortillas (or any gluten-free
tortillas of choice)

1 cup spinach or romaine

½ cup fire-roasted corn
(or sweet corn)

⅓ cup pico de gallo

Optional toppings: cilantro, avocado,
pickled onions

Jicama is an underrated root vegetable that I love for its hydrating crunch and punch of fiber. Get this: One cup of jicama provides nearly 7 grams of fiber and 43 percent of your recommended vitamin C daily intake! Similar to the texture of an apple, jicama makes for an unexpectedly satisfying, cool, and crispy taco filling. The ovulatory phase is all about light and refreshing meals, and these tacos are exactly that. Serve them up with some pico de gallo and pickled red onions! (Refer to page 99 to learn how to make your own pickled onions.)

Combine the jicama with the lime juice, chili powder, sea salt, and cayenne pepper, if using, in a medium bowl and toss to coat.

Heat a large frying over medium heat. Working in batches if necessary, cook each tortilla until warm and lightly browned, about 1 minute on each side.

To assemble, top each tortilla with spinach, jicama, corn, and pico de gallo, plus any additional toppings you desire. Serve immediately. Store any leftover jicama in an airtight container in the refrigerator for up to 3 days.

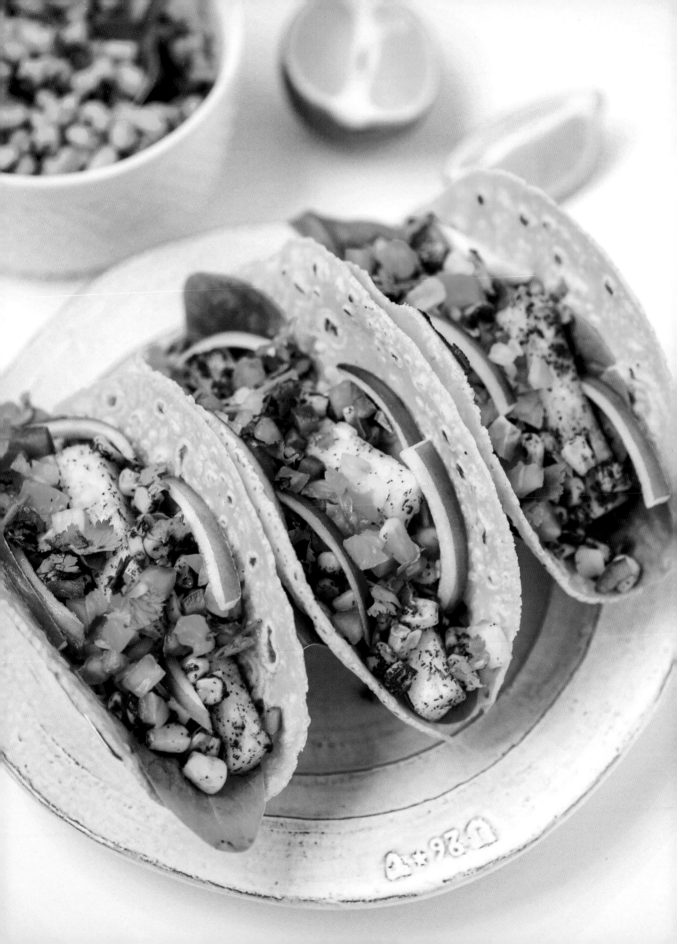

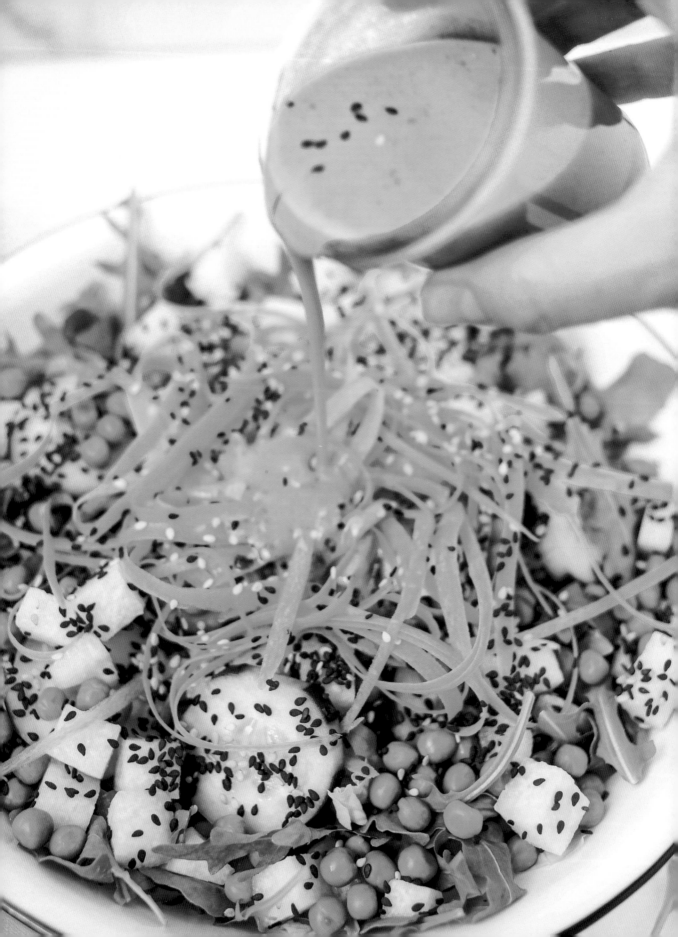

Arugula Sesame-Soy Salad

My husband calls this salad "restaurant quality." He's a total foodie and my biggest critic, so I will take the compliment! Arugula is the stand-out here with its clean peppery flavor, which pairs perfectly with the spicy sesame soy vinaigrette. It's also a cruciferous veggie, which we know has estrogen-detoxifying properties, perfect for the ovulatory and luteal phases. Cucumbers and jicama bring a nice crunch and lighten up the full-bodied flavors. Sprinkle in quinoa or some dried fruit like apricots for a sweet touch.

Combine the arugula, romaine, carrots, cucumber, peas, jicama, sesame seeds, and any optional add-ins in a large bowl.

Combine all the ingredients for the dressing in a small blender and blend until smooth. To serve immediately, pour the dressing over the salad and toss to mix. Divide among four plates and sprinkle each serving with extra sesame seeds. You can also refrigerate the salad and the dressing in separate airtight containers for up to 2 days; toss together immediately before serving.

SERVES: 4

SALAD

4 cups arugula

1 cup chopped romaine

2 large carrots, shaved

½ cucumber, chopped

½ cup green peas

½ cup cubed jicama

2 tablespoons sesame seeds (I used a mix of white and black), plus extra for sprinkling

Optional add-ins: quinoa, dried apricots

SESAME-SOY VINAIGRETTE

2 tablespoons filtered water

2 tablespoons tamari

2 tablespoons olive oil

1 tablespoon sesame oil

1 tablespoon rice vinegar

1 tablespoon pure maple syrup

Juice of 1 lime

½ teaspoon sea salt

½ teaspoon black pepper

Pinch of crushed red pepper flakes (optional)

Crunch Monster Summer Salad with Green Goddess Dressing

SERVES: 4

SALAD

2 bunches romaine, chopped

1 cup shredded green cabbage
(or purple cabbage)

1 bulb fennel, sliced (trim off the stalks
and save for a soup or broth)

½ cucumber, chopped

½ bell pepper, chopped

¼ cup sunflower seeds

¼ cup fresh mint, chopped

2 tablespoons chopped red onion

Optional add-ins: hemp seeds,
lentils, chickpeas

GREEN GODDESS DRESSING

½ cup tahini

½ cup filtered water

½ cup fresh cilantro

½ cup fresh parsley

2 green onions, roughly chopped

2 tablespoons apple cider vinegar

1 tablespoon pure maple syrup

Juice of 1 lime

1 teaspoon sea salt

¾ teaspoon black pepper

Let's set something straight: not every salad has to be stuffed with kale or dark greens. There are lots of other crunchy, hydrating lettuces out there, and this phase is the time to feast on them! This salad delivers the perfect flavor combination with green goddess dressing, mint, fennel, crunchy cucumber, sunflower seeds, and more. It's refreshing, light, creamy, and crunchy, yet hearty enough to have as a lunch salad. Feel free to add some hemp seeds, lentils, or chickpeas for extra protein.

Combine the romaine, green cabbage, fennel, cucumber, bell pepper, sunflower seeds, mint, red onion, and any optional add-ins in a large bowl.

Combine all the ingredients for the dressing in a small blender and blend until smooth and creamy.

To serve immediately, pour the dressing over the salad, toss to mix, and divide among four plates. You can also refrigerate the salad and the dressing in separate airtight containers for up to 3 days; toss together immediately before serving.

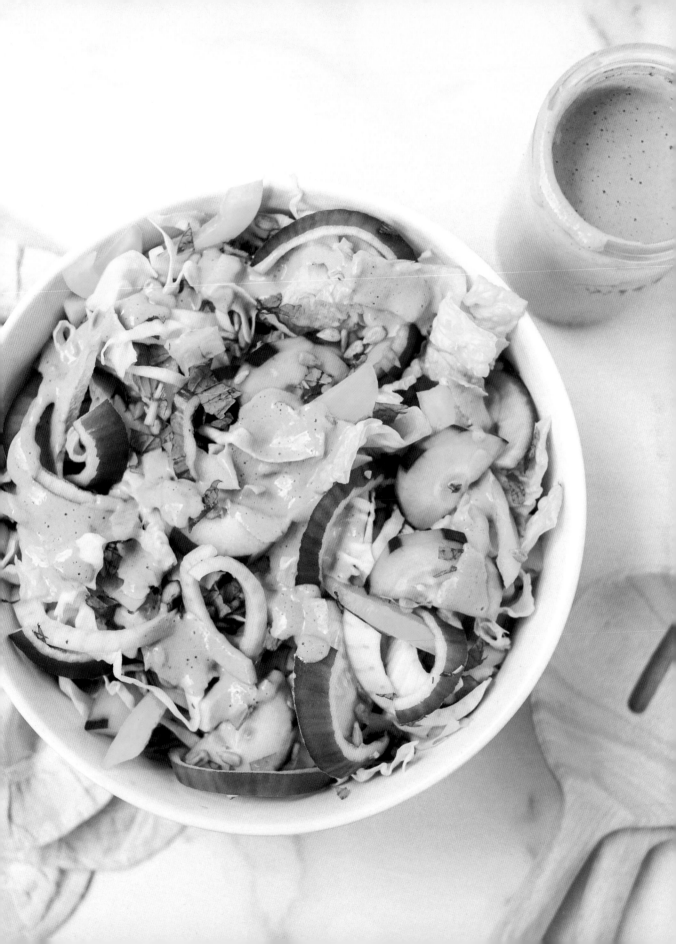

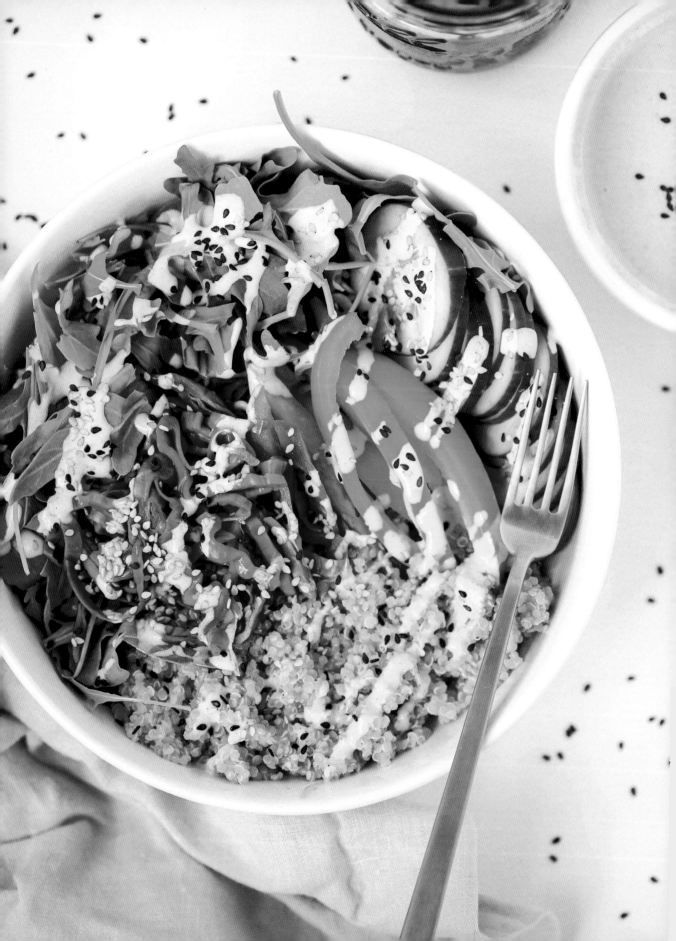

Tahini Buddha Bowl

I love mixing in crunchy raw veggies with quinoa, greens, and the creamiest tahini sauce for this beautiful buddha bowl. It's simple, flavorful, and full of colorful fiber and protein-rich quinoa. The beauty of ovulatory recipes is incorporating raw veggies to help increase glutathione, a powerful antioxidant that aids in liver detoxification. You can use any type of green lettuce or raw veggie combo you like, but I chose arugula, cucumber, bell peppers, and pickled purple cabbage for a nice balance. The rich tahini sauce brings it all together.

Combine the quinoa and vegetable broth in a medium saucepan over medium-high heat. Bring to a boil, then reduce the heat to low, cover, and simmer for 15 minutes, or until all the water is absorbed.

Combine all the ingredients for the quick-pickled cabbage in a small bowl, and make sure the cabbage is fully submerged in the liquid. Let sit for at least 20 minutes at room temperature while you prepare the rest of the recipe. If making ahead, store in the refrigerator after 20 minutes.

Combine all the ingredients for the tahini sauce in a small bowl and whisk together until smooth and creamy. Store in the refrigerator until ready to use.

To assemble the bowls, divide the arugula between two bowls, and top with the pickled cabbage, cucumber, bell pepper, quinoa, and sesame seeds. Drizzle each bowl with the tahini sauce and serve. Store any leftovers in an airtight container in the refrigerator for up to 3 days.

SERVES: 2

BOWL

½ cup quinoa

1 cup low-sodium vegetable broth (or filtered water)

3–4 cups arugula

½ cucumber, thinly sliced

½ bell pepper, thinly sliced

2 tablespoons sesame seeds

QUICK-PICKLED CABBAGE

1 cup very thinly sliced red cabbage (I use a mandoline slicer)

½ cup apple cider vinegar

½ cup filtered water

½ teaspoon sea salt

½ teaspoon coconut sugar

SIMPLE TAHINI SAUCE

¼ cup tahini

¼ cup filtered water

Juice of ½ lemon

1 teaspoon pure maple syrup

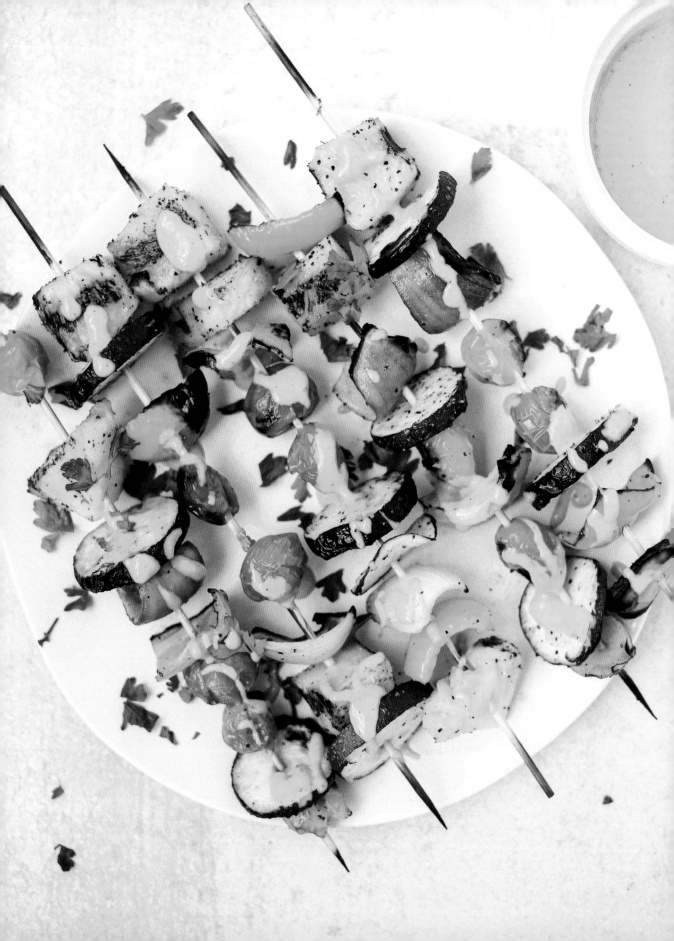

Prep Time: 15 minutes   **Cook Time:** 15 minutes   **Total Time:** 30 minutes

Spicy Grilled Veggie Kabobs with Tahini Turmeric Chili Sauce

Grilled kabobs are the ultimate summertime meal! If you don't have a grill, you can always use a grill pan and get the same effect! The charred grill taste is a nice change of flavor from your typical steamed or roasted veggies. The tasty Tahini Turmeric Chili Sauce has the most beautiful golden hue that adds a pop of color while providing anti-inflammatory properties from the curcumin in turmeric! Serve with a side of quinoa.

Combine the pineapple, cherry tomatoes, zucchini, bell pepper, and red onion in a large bowl. Add the coconut oil, sea salt, black pepper, and red pepper flakes, if using, and stir to mix until all veggies are coated.

Combine all the ingredients for the sauce in a small blender, starting with 1 tablespoon of water. (Or combine all the ingredients in a small bowl and whisk by hand.) Blend until smooth and creamy, adding up to 1 tablespoon more water until you reach the desired consistency. Set aside.

Carefully thread the veggies onto skewers. You should have 8–9 skewers in all. Preheat the grill to medium-high heat. Make sure to oil the grill grates to prevent sticking. Place the skewers directly on the grill and cook, rotating every few minutes, for a total of 10–15 minutes, until veggies are tender and charred on all sides.

To serve, remove the veggies from the skewers, divide among plates, and drizzle with the Tahini Turmeric Chili Sauce. Serve the veggies alongside some quinoa and greens. For leftovers, remove the veggies from the skewers and store in an airtight container in the refrigerator for up to 3 days.

SERVES: 3–4

KABOBS

2 cups cubed fresh pineapple

1 ½ cups cherry tomatoes

1 zucchini, sliced

1 bell pepper, cubed

½ red onion, cubed

2 tablespoons melted coconut oil

½ teaspoon sea salt

½ teaspoon black pepper

¼ teaspoon red pepper flakes (optional)

TAHINI TURMERIC CHILI SAUCE

3 tablespoons tahini

2 tablespoons olive oil

2 tablespoons chili paste

1 tablespoon sriracha

1–2 tablespoons filtered water

Juice of 2 limes

½ teaspoon ground turmeric

¼ teaspoon black pepper

¼ teaspoon ground cayenne pepper

Cilantro and Pistachio Pesto Quinoa

SERVES: 4

QUINOA MIXTURE

1 cup quinoa

2 cups filtered water

1 tablespoon coconut oil

1 small yellow squash, chopped

1 small zucchini, chopped

¼ cup pistachios

CILANTRO PESTO

1 cup packed fresh cilantro, plus extra for garnish

¼ cup nutritional yeast

3 tablespoons pistachios

1 clove garlic, minced

½ cup filtered water

2 tablespoons olive oil

Juice of ½ lemon, plus extra for squeezing

1 teaspoon pure maple syrup

½ teaspoon sea salt

¼ teaspoon red pepper flakes (optional)

This quinoa salad is a simple meal-prepping and phase-friendly dish. I love pesto because it can be made with so many different herbs. I chose cilantro for its bright, earthy flavor, but feel free to swap in parsley or basil, or a mix of the two. The fun twist here is the pistachios for their decadent flavor and array of nutrients, including vitamin B6, copper, and fiber.

Combine the quinoa and water in a medium saucepan over medium-high heat. Bring to a boil. Stir in the coconut oil, then reduce the heat to low, cover, and simmer for 15 minutes, or until all the water is absorbed.

Meanwhile, place the yellow squash and zucchini in a steamer basket. Bring a small amount of water to boil in a saucepan, place the steamer basket in the saucepan, cover, and reduce the heat to medium-low to steam for 5–7 minutes, or until soft.

Combine all the ingredients for the pesto in a small blender or food processor and blend until smooth and creamy.

Combine the cooked quinoa, steamed veggies, and pistachios in a large bowl. Pour the pesto on top and mix well. To serve, divide among plates and top each serving with a fresh squeeze of lemon and a sprinkle of cilantro. Store leftovers in an airtight container in the refrigerator for up to 3 days.

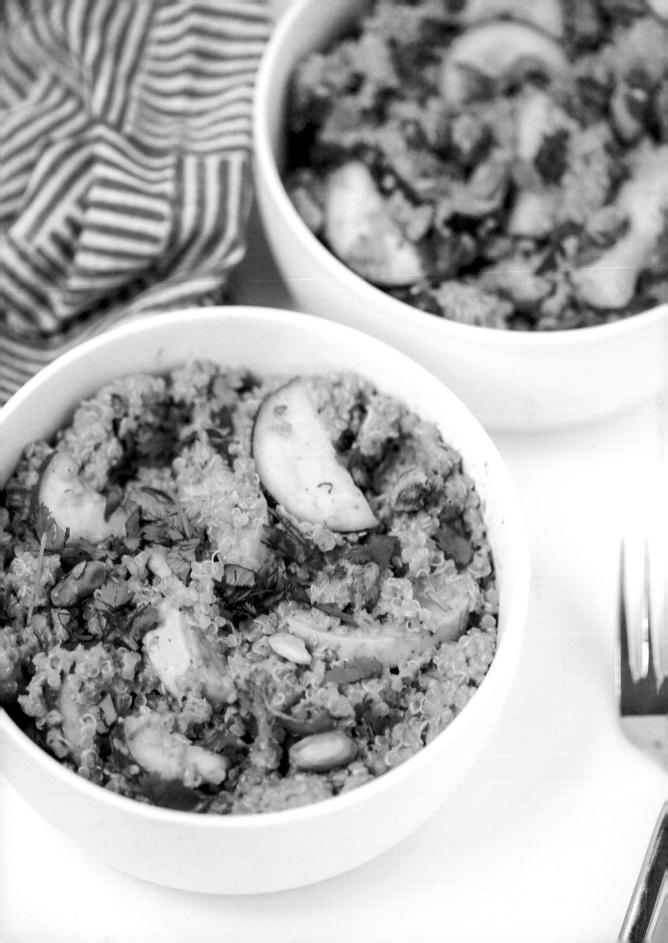

Sun-Dried Tomato Garden Burgers

MAKES: 8 BURGERS

1 tablespoon coconut oil, plus more as needed

⅓ yellow onion, chopped

1 bell pepper, chopped

1 clove garlic, minced

¾ teaspoon plus 1 pinch sea salt

½ teaspoon plus 1 pinch black pepper

¾ cup oat flour

2 tablespoons ground flaxseed

2 tablespoons nutritional yeast

1 tablespoon ground cumin

⅓ cup chopped parsley

⅓ cup sun-dried tomatoes

2 (15-ounce) cans great northern beans, drained and rinsed

Optional toppings: lettuce, vegan mayonnaise, tomato, onions

Everyone needs a go-to homemade veggie burger recipe! These are a staple in my rotation as they're veggie forward, filling, and so easy for meal prep. I eat them over a salad, in a sandwich, or in burger form with all the fixings. Thanks to the ground flaxseed, mashed white beans, and oat flour, these garden burgers are not too dense and do not fall apart. Sun-dried tomatoes add a sweet and tart flavor while providing vitamin C, vitamin B6, iron, and magnesium. Meanwhile, the great northern beans pack in fiber, protein, calcium, and iron. I cook the patties all at once so I can have them ready for lunches and dinners throughout the week. Yum!

Heat the coconut oil in a medium frying pan over medium-high heat. Add the onion and sauté until it turns translucent, 4–5 minutes. Add the bell pepper and garlic, plus a pinch each of sea salt and black pepper, and cook for 3 more minutes. Turn off the heat.

Combine the oat flour, flaxseed, nutritional yeast, cumin, and the remaining ¾ teaspoon sea salt and ½ teaspoon black pepper in a food processor. Blend until well combined. Transfer this dry mixture to a large bowl and stir in the chopped parsley.

Place the sun-dried tomatoes in the food processor and blend/pulse until shredded into tiny pieces, about the size of bacon bits. Transfer to the bowl with the dry mixture. Place the great northern beans in the food processor and blend until lightly mashed, with a few beans still intact for texture. Add the beans to the dry mixture, then add the sautéed onion and veggie mixture. Set the pan used to cook the veggies aside; do not clean it out.

Wet your hands and use them to mix everything in the bowl together, then form the mixture into 8 patties. Lay them flat on a plate and cover with plastic wrap.

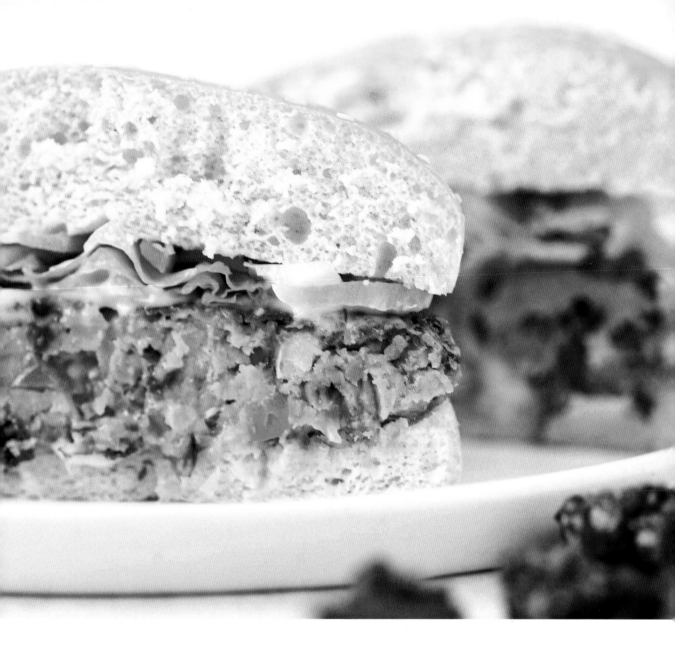

Refrigerate the patties for 20 minutes to set. This step helps the patties to firm up and hold together when cooked.

When ready to cook, remove the patties from the refrigerator. Heat the same frying pan you used to cook the veggies over medium heat. You may need to add a little more coconut oil. Add the patties to the hot pan, working in batches if necessary, and cook until golden brown, 4–5 minutes on each side.

Serve on a bun or over a salad with any of the optional toppings. Store leftovers in an airtight container in the refrigerator for up to 4 days.

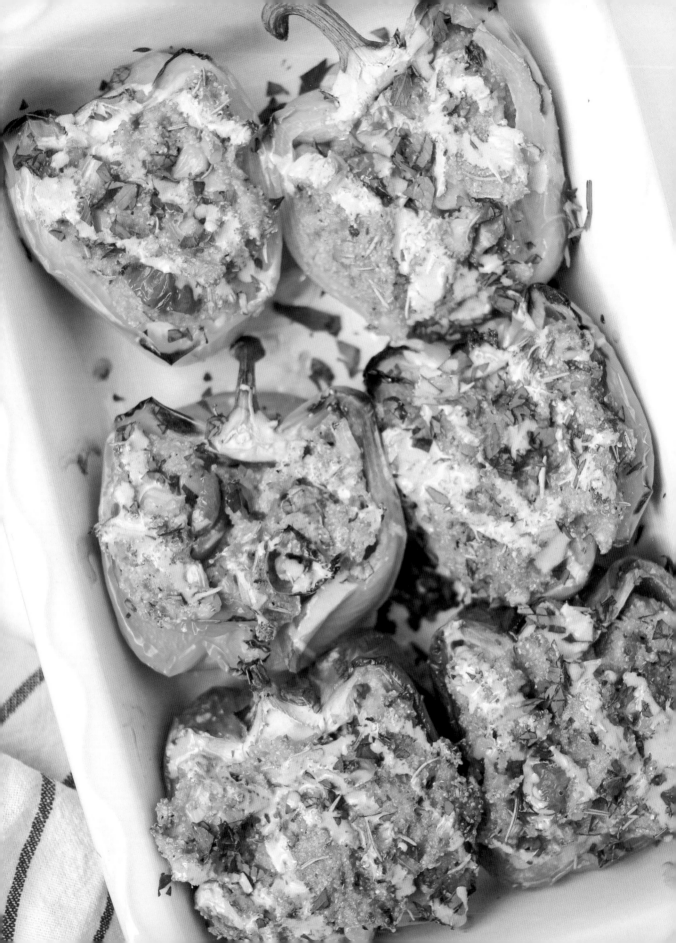

Amaranth and Veggie Stuffed Bell Peppers

Stuffed bell peppers feel like healthy comfort food to me. They are colorful and nourishing—my favorite kind of meal! Like many of the recipes in this phase, this one is rich in vitamin C, a powerful antioxidant that helps decrease oxidative damage, which is particularly important during ovulation for the health of your eggs. The peppers have a cozy rosemary flavor, and the juicy tomatoes bring an acidic brightness and keep the filling from drying out while roasting in the oven. You can always use quinoa instead of amaranth, if you prefer. I like to serve these with a side of salad, preferably the Crunch Monster Salad!

SERVES: 3

1 cup amaranth, rinsed well

2 cups low-sodium vegetable broth

½ cup cornmeal

1 tablespoon avocado oil

½ white onion, diced

1 cup finely chopped celery

½ cup quartered cherry tomatoes

1 cup sweet canned corn, drained and rinsed

1 clove garlic, minced

Pinch of sea salt and black pepper

1 ½ tablespoons chopped dried rosemary

3 bell peppers, halved, seeds removed

2 tablespoons chopped fresh parsley, for topping

It's really important to rinse off the amaranth first! I do this using a nut milk bag because the amaranth grain is so teeny.

Preheat the oven to 400°F. Line a baking sheet with parchment paper.

In a small saucepan, combine the amaranth and vegetable broth. Bring to a boil, then reduce the heat to a simmer, cover, and simmer for 20 minutes until water is absorbed. Turn off the heat and stir in the cornmeal. Set aside.

Heat the avocado oil in a medium frying pan over medium-high heat. Add the onion and sauté until it turns translucent, 4–5 minutes. Add the celery, cherry tomatoes, corn, garlic, and a pinch each of sea salt and black pepper. Cook for 4–5 more minutes, or until the veggies are softened. Turn off the heat.

Stir the veggies into the cooked amaranth. Lay the bell peppers cut side up on the lined baking sheet and spoon the amaranth-veggie mixture into each bell pepper. Bake on the center rack for 30 minutes.

Remove from the oven and let the peppers cool for a few minutes before serving. To serve, place two pepper halves on each plate and top with a sprinkle of fresh parsley. Store leftovers in an airtight container in the refrigerator for up to 3 days.

Yellow Lentil and Creamy Corn Chowder

SERVES: 4

¾ cup yellow lentils (also called split yellow mung beans)

2 tablespoons coconut oil

½ yellow onion

3 stalks celery, chopped

1 small zucchini, chopped

1 clove garlic, minced

1 teaspoon ground turmeric

1 teaspoon sea salt

½ teaspoon black pepper

1 ½ cups sweet corn (thawed if frozen)

2 cups filtered water (or low-sodium vegetable broth)

1 cup coconut milk

Optional toppings: crumbled crackers, red pepper flakes, green onion

Mildly sweet with a comforting coconut flavor, this chowder is one of my favorite recipes in this phase. Split yellow mung beans (or mung dal) are a traditional Ayurvedic-cleansing food and are known for their easy digestibility and soft texture. They're high in fiber and protein to help satiate you while the turmeric is helping to decrease inflammation. This is perfect to make in the fall or winter during ovulation because it feels summery but is also warming. Serve with toast or crackers!

Soak the lentils in water for 20 minutes, then rinse, drain, and set aside.

Heat the coconut oil in a large pot over medium heat. Add the onion and sauté for 3–4 minutes. Stir in the celery, zucchini, and garlic. Sauté for 3–4 minutes more. Stir in the ground turmeric, sea salt, and black pepper and cook for 2 more minutes, then stir in the sweet corn, water, coconut milk, and soaked lentils. Bring to a slow boil, then cover and reduce the heat to simmer for 20 minutes.

Divide the soup among four bowls, sprinkle with any optional toppings, and serve. Store leftovers in an airtight container in the refrigerator for up to 3 days or freeze for up to 2 months.

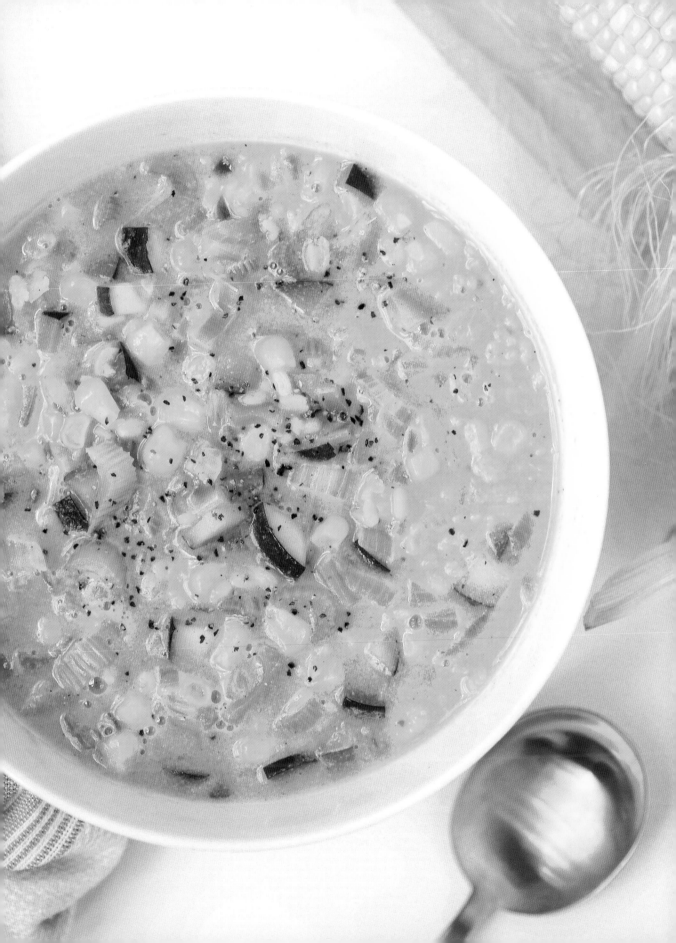

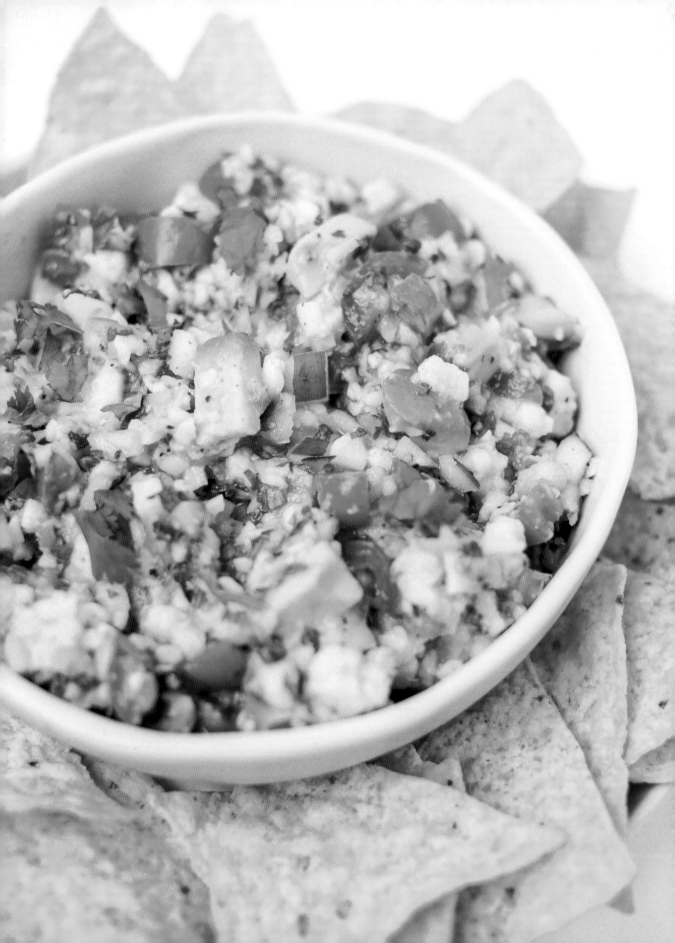

Prep Time: 10 minutes   Total Time: 10 minutes

Coconut Ceviche

Who would have thought that coconut meat would make the perfect substitute for seafood in ceviche? It mimics the texture like nothing else. I love bringing this to parties as an appetizer and not telling anyone it's vegan—it's always a hit! The mix of lemon and lime juice is essential for that bright acidity, while the coconut meat brings a slightly sweet flavor. I had to order coconut meat online (if only I had fresh coconuts in my backyard!), but some grocery stores carry canned coconut meat. This tasty snack is even better with tortilla chips!

Combine the coconut meat, cilantro, red onion, jalapeño, lime juice, and lemon juice in a food processor. Blend until finely chopped (do not over blend—it does not have to be perfect). Transfer to a small bowl and stir in the tomatoes, avocado, sea salt, black pepper, garlic powder, and dulse flakes, if using. Mix until well combined. Serve with tortilla chips. Store leftovers in an airtight container in the refrigerator for up to 2 days.

SERVES: 2–3

1 ½ cups fresh coconut meat (canned or fresh)

¾ cup fresh cilantro

2 tablespoons red onion, chopped

½ jalapeño, or more to taste

Juice of 1 lime

Juice of ½ lemon

½ cup chopped tomatoes

½ large ripe avocado (or 1 small avocado), cubed

½ teaspoon sea salt

½ teaspoon black pepper

¼ teaspoon garlic powder

1–2 teaspoons dulse flakes (optional; for fish taste)

Gluten-free tortilla chips, for serving

Sunflower Seed Snacking Spread

SERVES: 2–3

¾ cup sunflower seeds

2 large carrots, shredded

¾ cup parsley

½ shallot

1 clove garlic, minced

Juice of 1 lemon

3 tablespoons olive oil

2 tablespoons filtered water

2 tablespoons nutritional yeast

1 teaspoon paprika

½ teaspoon sea salt

½ teaspoon black pepper

½ teaspoon pure maple syrup

⅛ teaspoon ground cayenne pepper (optional)

This recipe is super versatile—spread it on crackers or toast, use it as a filling in a wrap, or serve it with fresh veggies as an appetizer or yummy snack. Lots of fresh parsley, veggies, citrus, and spices make this a delicious snack! Did you know soaking nuts and seeds (in this case, sunflower seeds) improves their nutrients and makes them more bioavailable by reducing the levels of phytic acid? It's fascinating. Soaking is optional but recommended for digestibility. Sunflower seeds are a great source of fiber, vitamin E, and iron.

Soak the sunflower seeds in hot water for 10 minutes. Drain and rinse, then blend the sunflower seeds in a food processor until ground. Transfer to a bowl.

Place the carrots in the food processor and blend until finely ground. Return the sunflower seeds to the food processor and add all the remaining ingredients. Blend until well combined and the texture resembles a dip or spread, scraping down the sides as needed.

Transfer to a small bowl and serve with crackers or veggies, or use as a spread in a sandwich or wrap. Store leftovers in an airtight container in the refrigerator for up to 2 days.

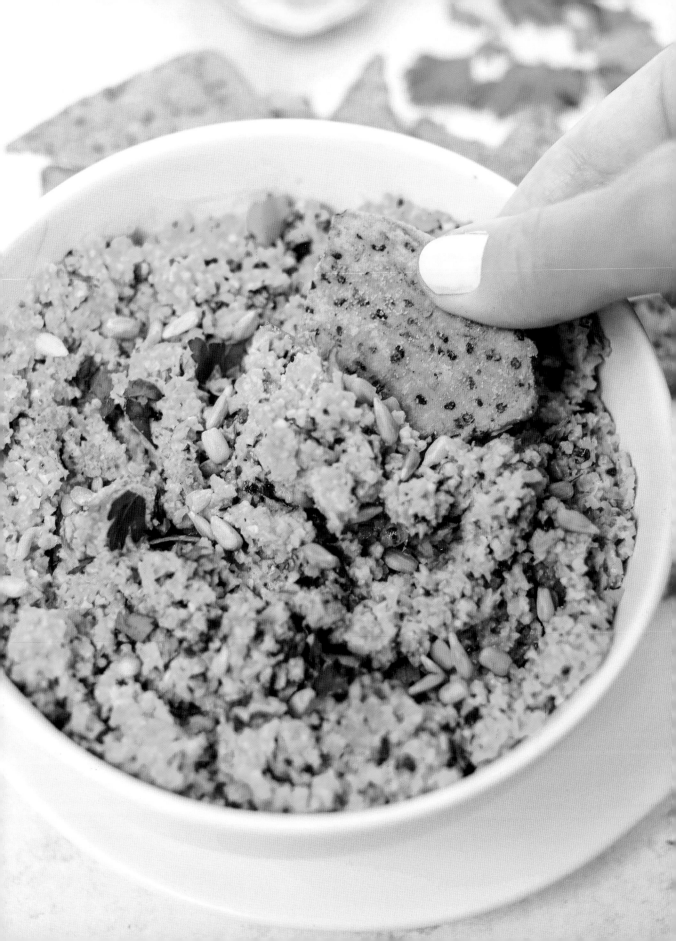

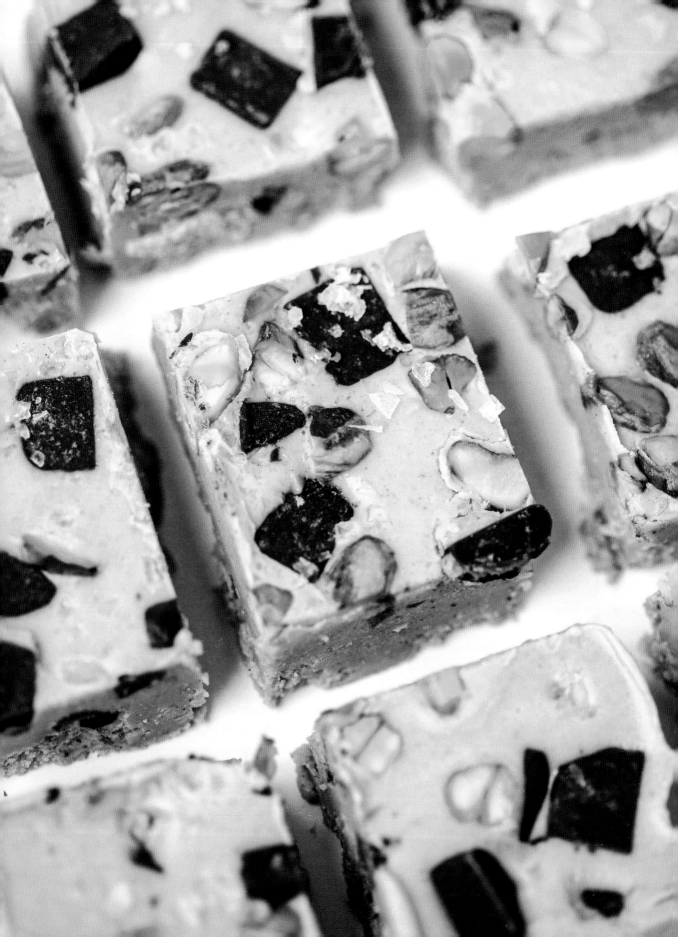

Prep Time: 5 minutes   **Freeze Time:** 30 minutes   **Total Time:** 35 minutes

Salted Pistachio Tahini Freezer Fudge

This sweet and salty no-bake freezer fudge tastes like cookie dough and makes for the yummiest summer treat. I devour anything with tahini. It's so rich and decadent, and it's especially delicious in fudge form. With vegan chocolate chips, pistachios for a salty crunch, hints of vanilla, and Maldon salt flakes, the flavor is super unique and satisfying. The meltaway texture is everything you want a rich fudge to be!

Line a 7x5-inch baking dish (I use a glass Tupperware dish) with parchment paper.

Combine the tahini, melted coconut oil, maple syrup, liquid stevia, vanilla extract, and sea salt in a small mixing bowl and whisk together until smooth. Fold in half of the vegan chocolate chips and half of the pistachios.

Transfer the fudge to the lined baking dish. Sprinkle the remaining chocolate chips and pistachios on top. Freeze for 30 minutes.

To serve, sprinkle with fancy sea salt and cut into squares. Store leftovers in an airtight container in the freezer for up to 2 months.

MAKES: 12 SQUARES

1 cup tahini

¼ cup melted coconut oil

1 tablespoon pure maple syrup

1–2 dropperfuls liquid stevia (or 1 more tablespoon maple syrup)

1 teaspoon vanilla extract

¼ teaspoon Maldon sea salt, plus more for sprinkling on top (regular sea salt will also work)

3 tablespoons vegan chocolate chips

3 tablespoons pistachios

Pineapple Green Juice Ice Pops

MAKES: 8 POPSICLES

2 ripe bananas

2 cups kale (or spinach, for a less "green" taste)

1 cup fresh or frozen chopped pineapple

½-inch knob fresh ginger, peeled

½-inch knob fresh turmeric, peeled

1 cup coconut water

Juice of ½ lemon

1 teaspoon vanilla extract

1 teaspoon pure maple syrup

Pinch of sea salt

Here's your green juice in popsicle form! Frozen treats don't get much healthier than these pops. They are anti-inflammatory and high in vitamin C while also keeping you cool and hydrated. When I think about summer desserts, I envision yummy ice pops while sitting outside on the porch. All you do is blend the ingredients as if you were making a smoothie, pour into the molds, and freeze! If you don't have a popsicle mold, you can pour them into paper cups or an ice cube tray and add popsicle sticks before freezing.

Combine all the ingredients in a high-speed blender. Blend until smooth. Pour the liquid into eight popsicle molds and freeze for 4–6 hours. When the popsicles are fully frozen, run the molds under warm water for a few seconds to loosen them up. Remove the popsicles from the molds and serve immediately, or store in an airtight container in the freezer for up to 3 months.

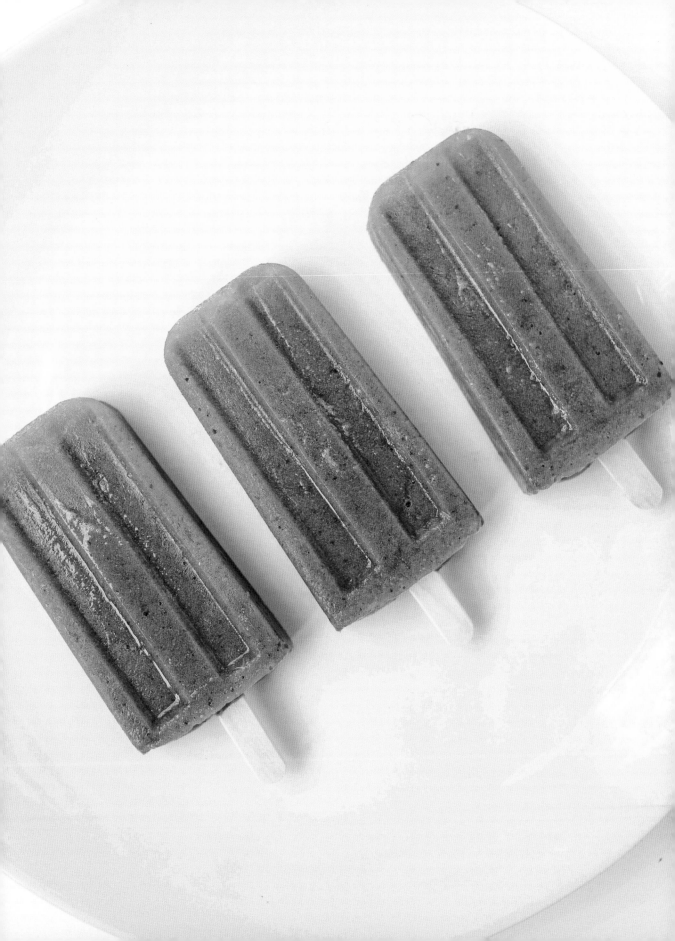

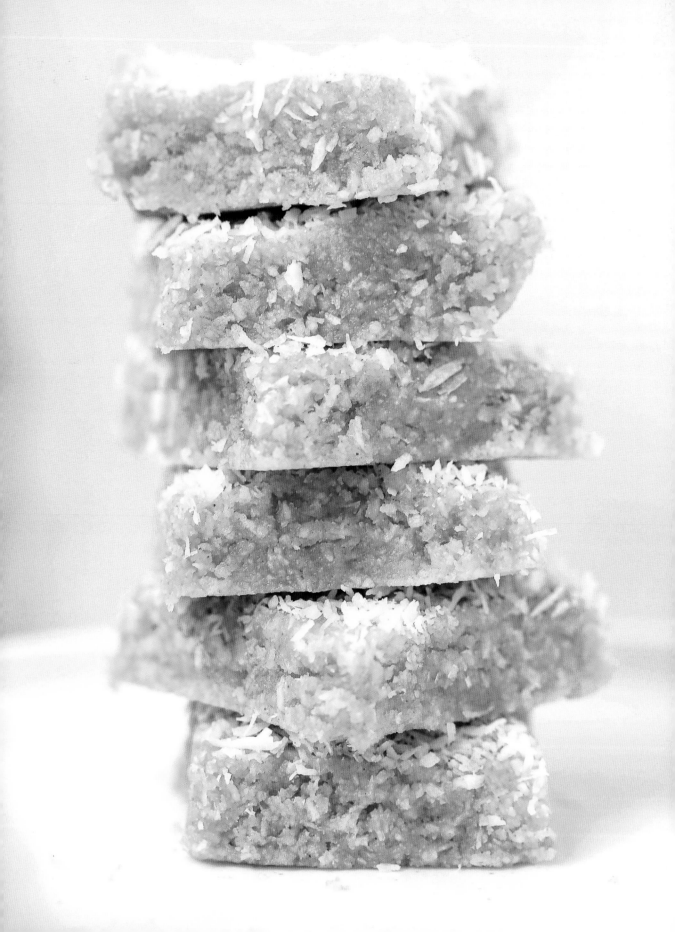

Prep Time: 5 minutes   **Cook Time:** 30 minutes   **Total Time:** 35 minutes

Peaches and Cream Millet Porridge

We know that the luteal phase is all about comforting, warming foods, so start your day off with this healthy version of peaches and cream oatmeal. It tastes like those oatmeal packets from childhood but has way less sugar! I chose millet, an ancient seed that's naturally gluten free, rich in B vitamins and magnesium, and has a mild, slightly sweet corn flavor. The vanilla protein powder adds flavor and helps slow the absorption of carbohydrates to keep your blood sugar stable. Pouring in a little extra liquid makes this porridge as creamy as can be.

SERVES: 2–3

1 ½ cups light coconut milk

1 ½ cups filtered water

1 cup millet, rinsed and drained (or gluten-free oats; if using oats reduce the cooking time to 10–15 minutes)

2 ripe peaches, sliced (or pears)

1 scoop vegan vanilla protein powder

1 tablespoon pure maple syrup

1 teaspoon vanilla extract

Pinch of sea salt

Optional toppings: almond butter, tahini, extra coconut milk, chopped dates, raisins, shredded coconut, sunflower seeds, chia seeds

Combine the coconut milk and water in a small saucepan and bring to a boil. (Be mindful and watch so it doesn't boil over.) Add the millet and reduce the heat to simmer, uncovered, for about 15 minutes, then add the sliced peaches and simmer for 10–15 minutes more. Once the millet is the consistency of creamy oatmeal, add the protein powder, maple syrup, vanilla extract, and sea salt and stir until smooth.

To serve, divide the porridge among bowls and sprinkle with any optional toppings. Store leftovers in an airtight container in the refrigerator for up to 2 days.

Sweet Potato Pancakes

SERVES: 2

1 baked sweet potato

2 ripe bananas, mashed

½ cup oat flour

1 teaspoon baking powder

½ teaspoon ground cinnamon

Pinch of sea salt

1 tablespoon coconut oil, plus more if needed

Optional toppings: sliced bananas, pears, pecans or walnuts, coconut yogurt, pure maple syrup

Sweet potatoes are known for their vibrant orange color and comforting texture and taste. Why not try them for breakfast? These pancakes are naturally sweet from the mashed banana and sweet potato, so you don't need to add any sweetener to the batter. They are so simple and scrumptious. Sweet potatoes are a complex carbohydrate, so these won't spike your blood sugar like your average pancakes. They're also high in vitamin B6, which can help reduce PMS symptoms (especially moodiness!) as well as Vitamin A in the form of beta-carotene, which gives them their beautiful orange hue. I recommend prepping your sweet potato by baking it the night before so you can whip these up quickly in the morning.

Peel the sweet potato and bananas and mash them together in a medium bowl. Stir in the oat flour, baking powder, cinnamon, and sea salt, and mix to combine.

Heat the coconut oil in a large sauté pan over medium heat. Working in batches if necessary, scoop ¼ cup of the batter for each pancake and drop it into the pan, using the measuring cup to press the batter down into small, circular pancakes. Cook the pancakes for 4–5 minutes, then flip and cook another 4–5 minutes, or until nicely browned on each side. Add more coconut oil if needed between batches.

Divide the pancakes between two plates and serve with a side of fruit, a drizzle of maple syrup, and any other optional toppings. Store any leftovers in an airtight container in the refrigerator for up to 2 days; reheat in a little coconut oil in a pan over medium heat.

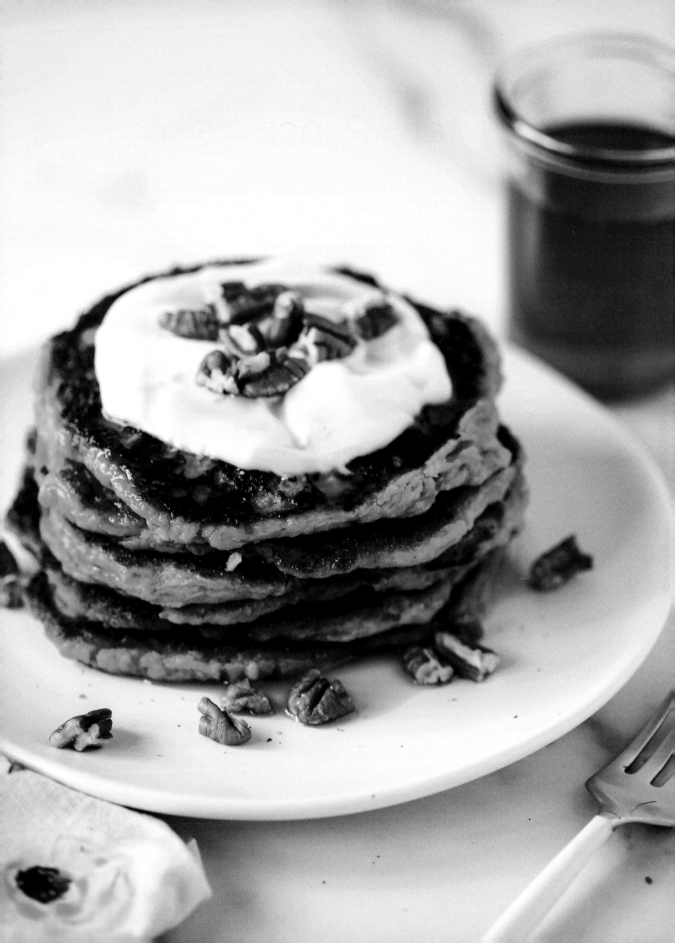

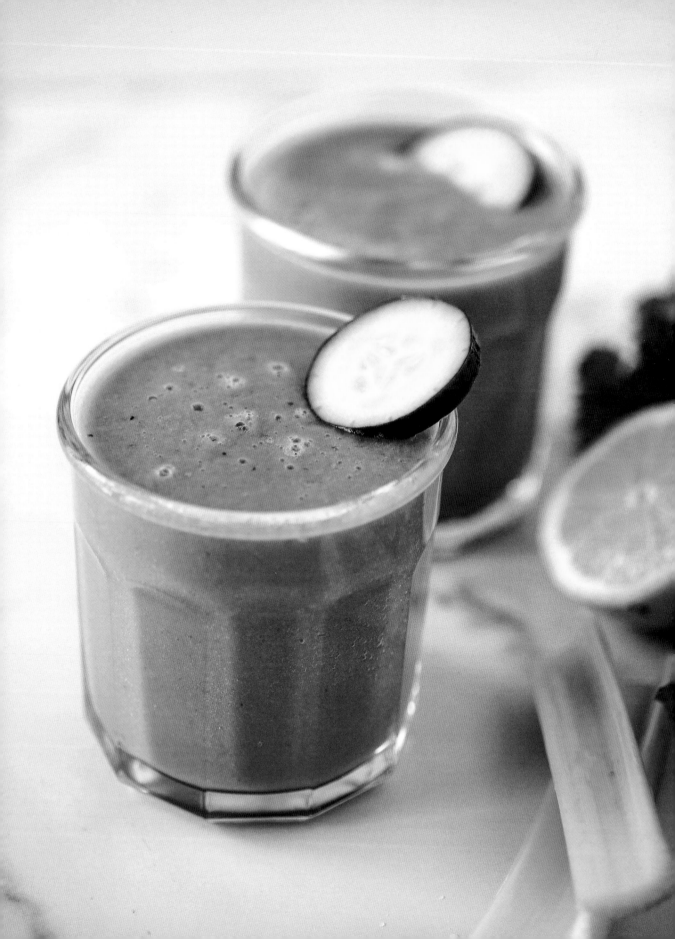

Estrogen Detox Green Smoothie

This is your ultimate liver-loving, hormone-loving detoxifying green smoothie. I drink this throughout my cycle because I crave it like crazy, but it's especially helpful in the ovulatory and luteal phases to help eliminate used-up estrogen. This simple smoothie is full of veggies with spices and a little fruit, but no added protein powder (adding protein powder will defeat the whole purpose of this smoothie and can cause bloating!). I recommend drinking it first thing in the morning on an empty stomach and then having some proteins and healthy fats about 30 minutes later—the Peaches and Cream Porridge or the Apple Un-Oatmeal are great options!

Combine all the ingredients in a high-speed blender. Blend until smooth. Serve immediately.

SERVES: 1

2 cups kale or spinach

1–2 stalks celery

½ cucumber

1 cup frozen mango

½ frozen banana

½ lemon (remove peel if not organic)

1-inch knob fresh ginger, peeled

1-inch knob fresh turmeric, peeled

1 small handful fresh cilantro

1 ½ cups filtered water

Apple Pie Un-Oatmeal

SERVES: 1

1 large apple, chopped

2 medjool dates, pitted and chopped

3 tablespoons shredded coconut

2 tablespoons chopped walnuts

2 tablespoons raisins (optional)

1 tablespoon chia seeds

1 teaspoon ground cinnamon

Juice of ½ lemon

2 tablespoons filtered water

1 tablespoon pure maple syrup (optional)

1 teaspoon vanilla extract

Optional toppings: granola, almond butter, raisins, hemp seeds

Who wants apple pie for breakfast? Because I swear, this combo tastes like an actual apple pie in a bowl! Warm apples infused with cinnamon plus vanilla, gooey dates, chewy raisins, brain-healthy walnuts, and shredded coconut make for the most delicious and comforting morning treat. It comes together faster than oatmeal, is packed with Vitamin C and fiber, and will make your whole house smell like fall in the best possible way. You can also turn this into a "cereal" by pouring in almond milk or your favorite plant-based milk.

Combine all the ingredients in a small saucepan over medium-low heat and stir. Cover and cook for 4–5 minutes, or until the apple is softened. Transfer to a bowl, sprinkle with any optional toppings, and serve. Store leftovers in an airtight container in the refrigerator for up to 2 days.

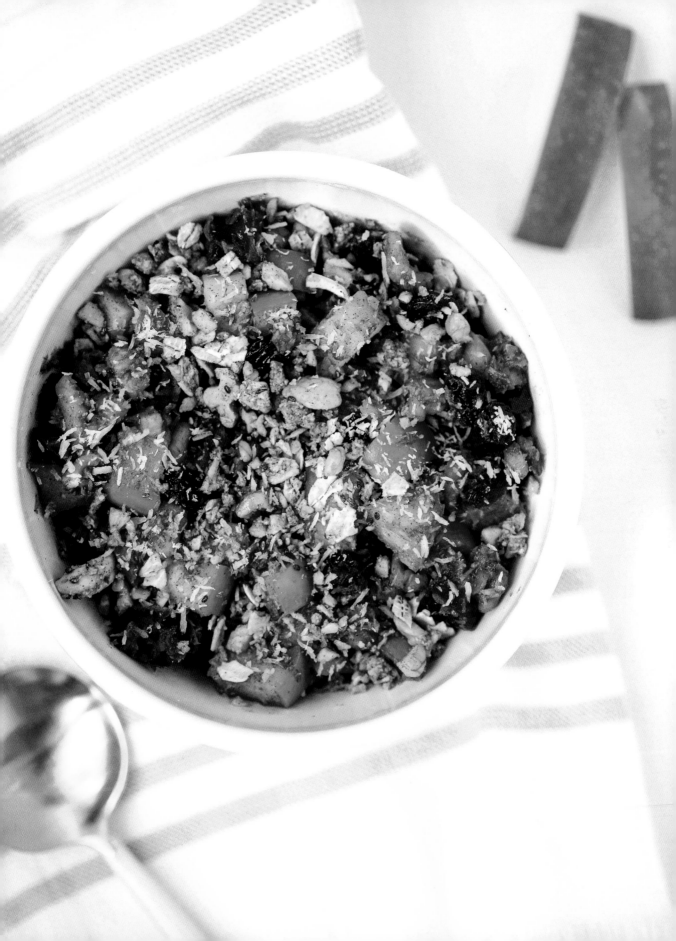

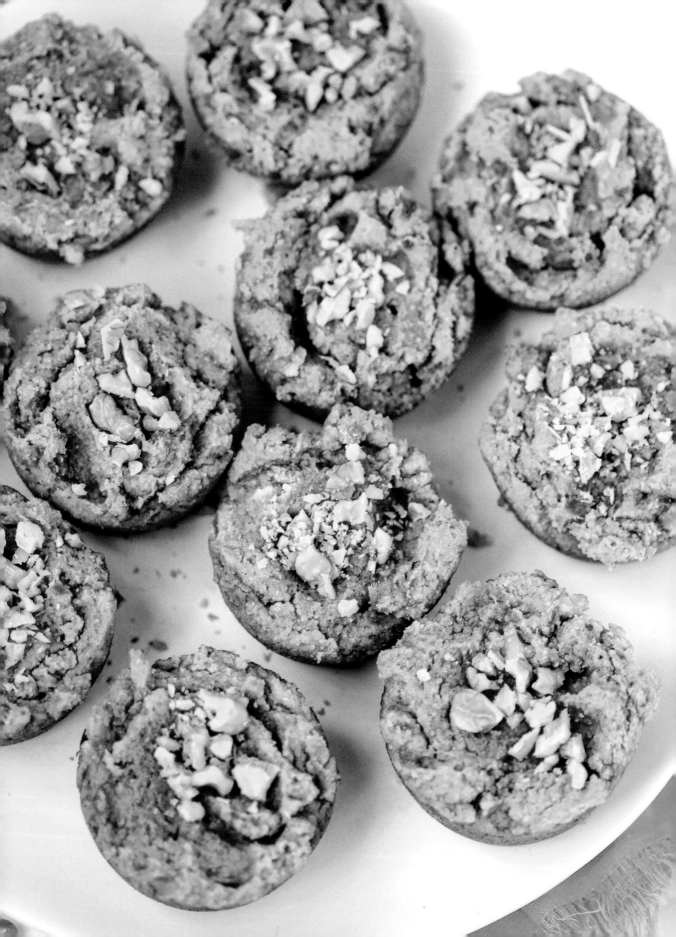

Gooey Banana Bread Muffins

Banana bread is a staple breakfast treat, and I love this vegan version in muffin form, which is easy to grab on the go! If you want to throw in some vegan chocolate chips, go for it, but I aimed to keep these low in sugar for happy hormones. Drizzle some raw almond butter on top for an extra hit of protein. These are made with almond flour, coconut flour, and hemp seeds for added fiber and healthy fats.

MAKES: 12 MUFFINS

1 ½ cups mashed banana (about 3 ripe bananas)

½ cup coconut milk

¼ cup melted coconut oil

¼ cup coconut sugar (or monk fruit sugar)

3 tablespoons ground flaxseed

3 tablespoons runny almond butter, plus more for drizzling

1 teaspoon vanilla extract

1 ½ cups almond flour

¾ cup coconut flour

2 teaspoons baking powder

1 teaspoon ground cinnamon

¼ cup hemp seeds (optional)

¼ cup walnuts (optional)

⅓ cup vegan chocolate chips (optional)

Preheat the oven to 350°F. Lightly grease a 12-cup muffin tin with coconut oil or line with muffin liners.

Place the bananas in a large mixing bowl and mash with a fork. Add the coconut milk, coconut oil, coconut sugar, ground flaxseed, almond butter, and vanilla extract and whisk together until smooth.

Stir in the almond flour, coconut flour, baking powder, and cinnamon. Then fold in the hemp seeds, walnuts, and vegan chocolate chips, if using.

Divide the batter evenly among the muffin cups. Bake for 17–20 minutes, or until the tops are golden brown and a toothpick inserted in the center of a muffin comes out clean. Let cool for a few minutes in the muffin pan, then remove from the pan, drizzle some almond butter on top, and serve. Store in an airtight container at room temperature for up to 3 days, or freeze for up to 3 months.

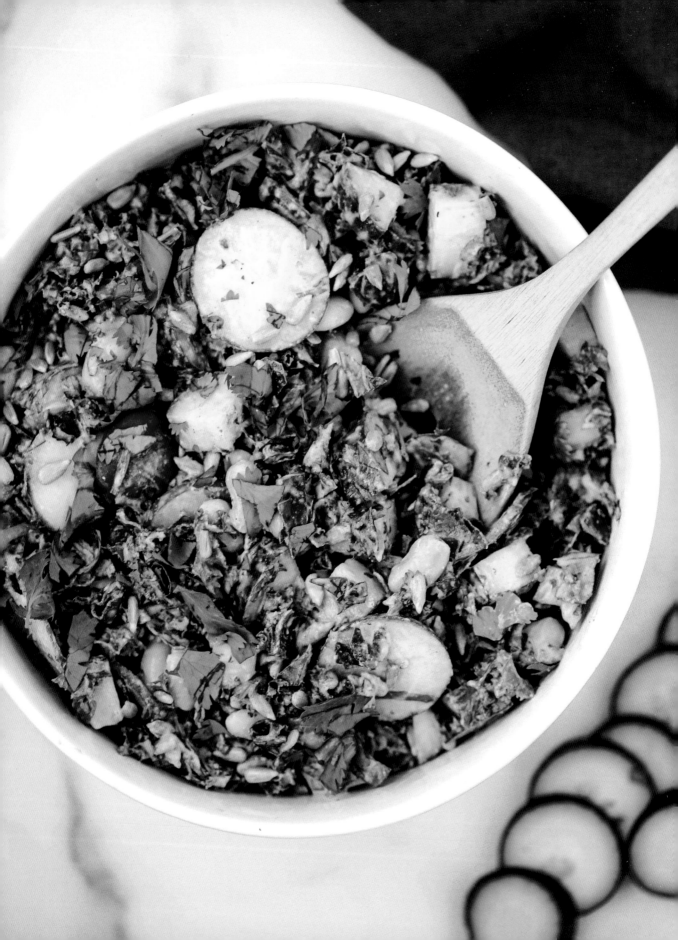

Prep Time: 15 minutes   **Total Time:** 15 minutes

Chopped Crunchy Kale Salad

The key to this salad is chopping the greens and veggies into small pieces so you can get a little bit of everything in each bite. I like to use salad scissors to keep it quick and easy. You really need a creamy, luscious dressing to balance out the tougher texture of kale, and this Tahini Dijon is heavenly. The cucumber and cabbage bring that perfect crunch you need for a chopped salad. I added white beans for protein, fiber, and iron and sunflower seeds for their selenium to support liver function and elimination of excess hormones!

Combine the kale, purple cabbage, great northern beans, cucumber, radishes, cilantro, mint, and sunflower seeds in a large salad bowl. Mix well.

Combine all the ingredients for the dressing in a small blender, starting with ¼ cup of the water. Blend until smooth, adding more water as needed to reach the desired consistency.

To serve immediately, pour the dressing over the salad and mix until well combined. Divide the salad among four plates, sprinkle with extra sunflower seeds, and serve. You can also refrigerate the salad and the dressing in separate airtight containers for up to 3 days; toss together immediately before serving.

SERVES: 4

SALAD

3 cups finely chopped kale

2 cups finely shredded purple cabbage

1 (15-ounce) can great northern beans, drained and rinsed

1 cucumber, chopped small

1 cup thinly sliced or finely chopped radishes

½ cup fresh chopped cilantro

⅓ cup fresh chopped mint

⅓ cup sunflower seeds, plus extra for sprinkling

Optional add-ins: Spicy "Honey" Mustard–Roasted Chickpeas (see page 187), roasted butternut squash, roasted sweet potato, roasted cauliflower

TAHINI DIJON DRESSING

⅓ cup runny tahini

¼–⅓ cup filtered water, as needed

2 tablespoons fresh lemon juice

2 teaspoons Dijon mustard

2 teaspoons pure maple syrup

1 ½ teaspoons tamari (or liquid aminos/coconut aminos)

Pinch of sea salt and black pepper

Baked Sweet Potato Falafel

SERVES: 4

FALAFEL

2 sweet potatoes

1 can chickpeas, drained and rinsed

½ red onion, chopped

¼ cup chopped cilantro

½ teaspoon ground cumin

½ teaspoon paprika

½ teaspoon sea salt

½ teaspoon black pepper

Juice of ½ lime

¼ cup oat flour

¼ cup sesame seeds, plus extra for sprinkling

EASY TAHINI SAUCE

¼ cup runny tahini

2 tablespoons filtered water, plus more as needed

Juice of ½ lemon

1 teaspoon pure maple syrup

If you're noticing a theme with sweet potatoes in the luteal phase, it's intentional! They are high in nutrients and grounding, which is exactly what we need in this phase. Plus, they are so versatile. This twist on falafel is baked instead of fried and made with mashed chickpeas and roasted sweet potato. I have to say I nailed the texture on these—they are soft and fluffy on the inside and firm on the outside, just like good falafel should be. Falafel is great for meal prepping because you can add it to any salad or bowl, eat them in a wrap, or all on their own. To save time, roast the sweet potatoes ahead of time.

Preheat the oven to 425°F and line a baking sheet with parchment paper.

Cut the sweet potatoes in half lengthwise (this helps them cook faster). Bake them in the oven for 30–35 minutes, or until fork-tender. Allow the sweet potatoes to cool slightly, then remove the skin.

Place the peeled sweet potatoes in a large bowl and mash well with a fork. Add the chickpeas and mash half of the chickpeas, leaving the other half whole for texture. Add the red onion, cilantro, cumin, paprika, sea salt, black pepper, and lime juice and mix. Mix in the oat flour and sesame seeds. You want the falafel mixture to hold together well but not be so sticky that it sticks to your hands. If it's too sticky, add 1–2 tablespoons more oat flour until you get the right consistency.

Using a cookie scoop or your hands, form golf ball-sized falafel balls and space them evenly on the lined baking sheet. I like to slightly flatten them out with my hands and sprinkle with more sesame seeds. You could also spray them with some olive oil cooking spray for an even crispier exterior.

Bake for 30–35 minutes, until golden brown.

Combine all the ingredients for the tahini sauce in a small bowl and whisk together until smooth and creamy, adding 1–2 tablespoons more water if your tahini is too thick.

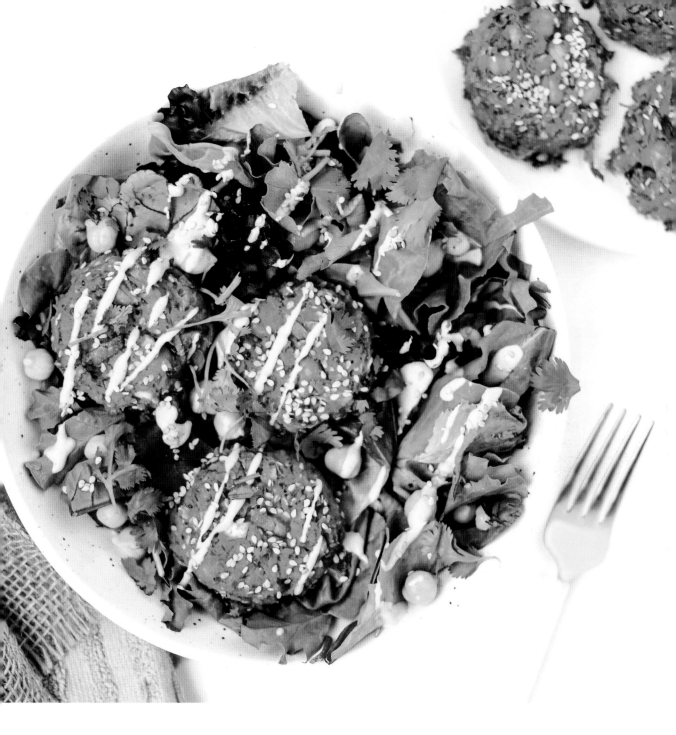

Serve the falafel immediately on their own with the tahini sauce, in wraps, or over salad. I like to serve mine over a bed of greens with purple cabbage and lots of tahini sauce. Store leftovers in an airtight container in the refrigerator for up to 4 days.

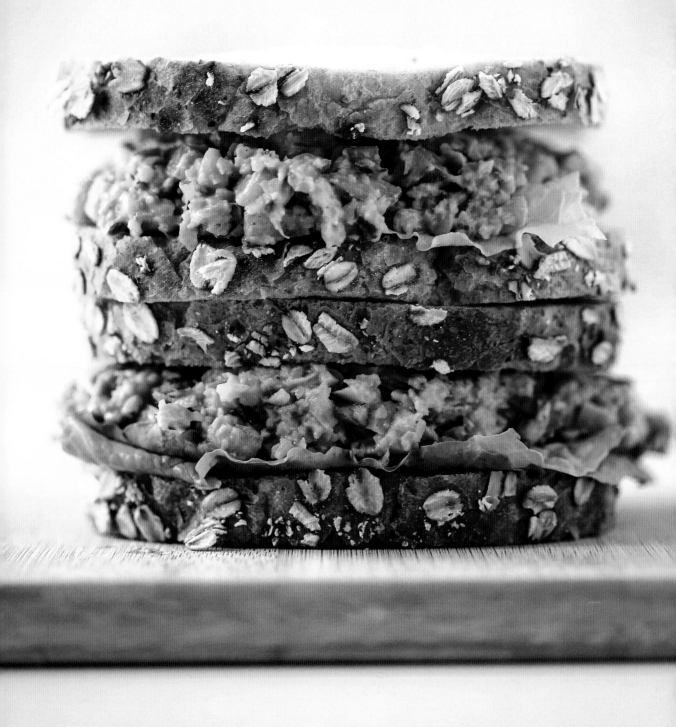

Mashed Chickpea Rainbow Salad

Mashed chickpea salads have been a go-to lunch for me ever since I went vegan. They are easy to prep ahead of time, and versatile to use throughout the week by layering over toast, serving on top of greens, or eating in a wrap. This particular recipe tastes better with time as the flavors blend and settle while in the refrigerator. Hearty and filling with plenty of fiber, fat, and protein, this salad will keep your blood sugar balanced and sugar cravings low. Feel free to pair it with avocado for extra healthy fats.

SERVES: 4

2 (15-ounce) cans chickpeas, drained and rinsed

1 cup chopped celery

1 cup shredded carrot

½ cup chopped bell pepper

½ cup shredded purple cabbage

½ cup chopped dill pickles

⅓ cup sunflower seeds

2 tablespoons red onion, minced

⅓ cup vegan mayonnaise

¼ cup Dijon mustard

2 tablespoons tahini

Juice of 1 lemon, plus extra for serving

Pinch of sea salt and black pepper

Place the chickpeas in a food processor and pulse until slightly mashed. Transfer them to a medium mixing bowl. Add the rest of the ingredients to the bowl and mix until well combined and creamy.

Taste test and adjust the amount of lemon, sea salt, and black pepper as needed. Divide the salad among four plates and serve with extra lemon. I like to serve this over lettuce on toast, or over a bed of greens. Store leftovers in an airtight container in the refrigerator for up to 4 days.

Prep Time: **10 minutes**   Cook Time: **35 minutes**   Total Time: **45 minutes**

Creamy Cauliflower Potato Soup

SERVES: 4

2 tablespoons avocado oil

½ yellow onion, chopped

4 cups cauliflower florets (1 head)

2 cloves garlic

3 cups Yukon gold potatoes, cubed

1 ½ teaspoons sea salt

1 teaspoon black pepper

1 teaspoon dried parsley

½ teaspoon ground mustard

2 bay leaves

3 cups low-sodium vegetable broth

1 cup canned coconut milk (or any plant-based milk)

⅓ cup nutritional yeast

Juice of ½ lemon

Optional toppings: green onion, cracked pepper, red pepper flakes

What's better than a creamy and hearty soup? I crave comfort foods in the luteal phase, and this recipe is a super-healthy way to satisfy that craving. The gold potatoes blended with cauliflower make for a luscious creamy base, while the bay leaves, nutritional yeast (packed with B vitamins), and spices add so much flavor. Eating any type of starch helps boost serotonin levels, which is why I'm a huge fan of potatoes of all kinds. Cooking and cooling potatoes creates resistant starch that ferments during digestion and sparks your good gut bacteria to go on a feeding frenzy. After breaking down the resistant starch, the bacteria start producing short-chain fatty acids, one of them being butyrate, which is known as a weight loss and inflammation-reducing compound. So now you have my permission to eat more potatoes—starting with this soup!

Heat the avocado oil in a large pot over medium heat. Add the onion and sauté for 3–4 minutes. Stir in the cauliflower and garlic and sauté for 5–6 minutes to soften slightly. Add the potatoes, sea salt, black pepper, dried parsley, ground mustard, and bay leaves. Then pour in the vegetable broth and coconut milk and stir.

Bring to a boil, then cover and reduce the heat to simmer for 25–30 minutes, or until the cauliflower and potatoes are fork-tender. Turn off the heat and stir in the nutritional yeast and lemon juice.

Remove the bay leaves. Using a hand immersion blender, carefully blend the soup until you reach the desired consistency. I prefer it really smooth and creamy, but feel free to leave pieces of cauliflower and potato for texture. You can also transfer the soup to a high-speed blender, working in batches if necessary, and blend until smooth. Be very careful and be sure to stop blending once in a while to let out the hot air and prevent a soup explosion!

To serve, divide the soup among bowls and sprinkle on any optional toppings. Store leftovers in an airtight container in the refrigerator for up to 3 days or freeze for up to 2 months.

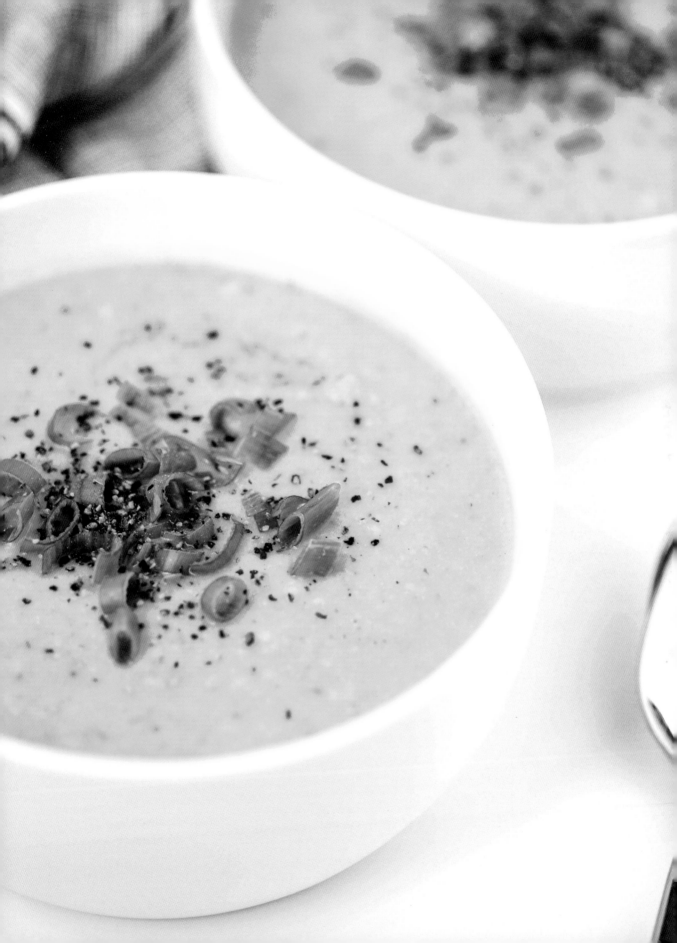

Harissa and Roasted Vegetable Nourish Bowl

SERVES: 2–3

BOWL

2 cups cubed butternut squash (about half of a small squash)

2 cups brussels sprouts, trimmed and halved

½ head cauliflower florets

⅓ red onion, diced

2 tablespoons avocado oil

½ teaspoon sea salt

½ teaspoon black pepper

4 cups chopped kale

1 (15-ounce) can chickpeas, drained and rinsed

Optional toppings: hemp seeds, sesame seeds

HARISSA SAUCE

1 cup roasted red peppers

2 Fresno chiles, ribs and stem removed

½ habanero pepper, rib and stem removed

2 cloves garlic

3 tablespoons olive oil

3 tablespoons fresh lemon juice (from about 1 ½ lemons)

2 teaspoons pure maple syrup

1 ½ teaspoons ground cumin

1 teaspoon ground coriander

1 teaspoon caraway seeds

1 teaspoon sea salt

½ teaspoon black pepper

This bowl is bright, spicy, nourishing, and all about the sauce. Harissa sauce is a spicy, slightly smoky hot sauce found in traditional North African and Moroccan cuisine. It's easy to blend, and you can adjust the spice level to your preference (start slow with those habaneros—you can always add more later!). The sauce has a stunning red-orange color and pairs so beautifully with roasted vegetables and chickpeas. I like the warmth of lightly steamed kale here, but you can opt for raw kale or any other green. Note: the sauce can also be used in rice dishes, on salads, or as a dip!

Preheat the oven to 400°F. Line a sheet pan with parchment paper.

Combine the butternut squash, brussels sprouts, cauliflower, and red onion in a large mixing bowl and toss with the oil, sea salt, and black pepper. Transfer the veggies to the lined sheet pan and spread out evenly. Bake for 30–35 minutes, or until squash is fork-tender.

Meanwhile, combine all the ingredients for the harissa sauce in a small blender and blend until smooth.

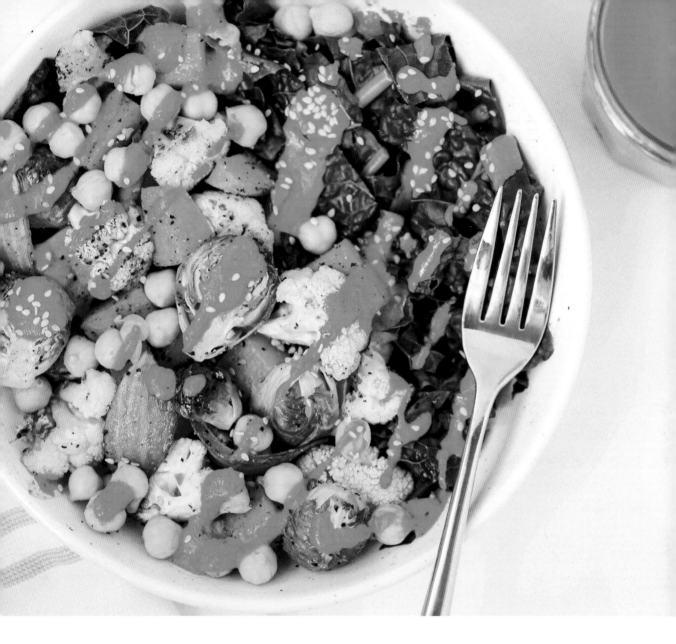

If desired, lightly steam the kale in a steamer basket over a pot of boiling water on the stove, covered, until slightly wilted and bright green. You can also leave the kale raw, if you prefer.

Once the veggies are done, allow them to cool slightly. To assemble, divide the kale, roasted veggies, and chickpeas among bowls. Then drizzle the harissa sauce over the top, add any optional toppings, and serve. If you have leftovers, store the sauce and veggies in separate airtight containers in the refrigerator for up to 3 days.

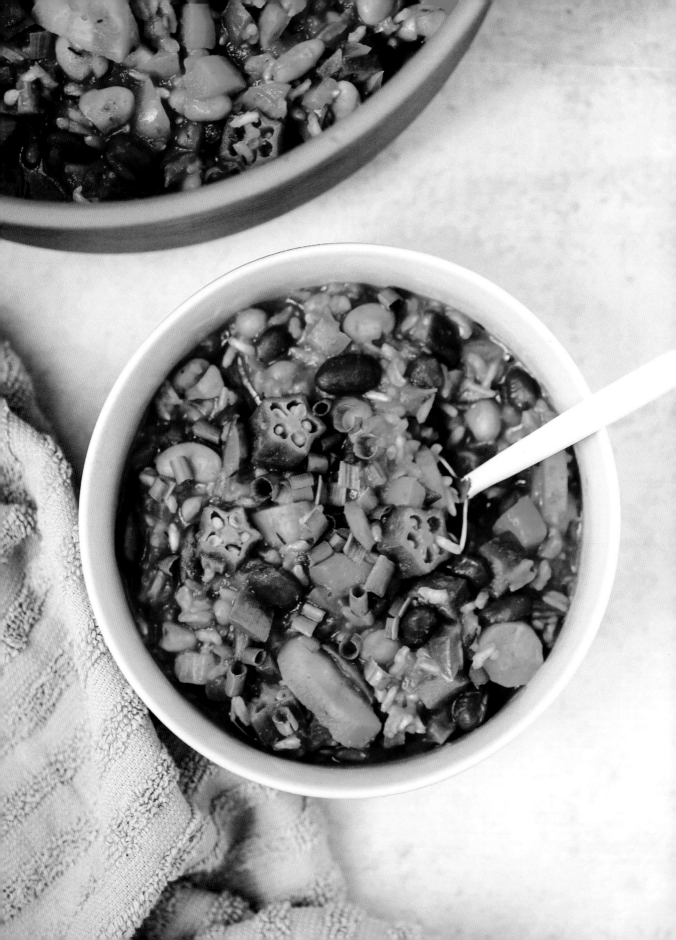

Prep Time: 10 minutes   **Cook Time:** 55 minutes   **Total Time:** 65 minutes

White Bean Jambalaya

A comforting and cheap one-pot meal, this dish has all the classic flavors of jambalaya with some minor twists to make it luteal-phase friendly. The tomato-infused broth is aromatic with smoky spices and herbs. Blend in hearty brown rice, a mix of kidney beans and white beans, and plenty of veggies. You can get creative with the veggies; I chose parsnips instead of carrots because they are phase-friendly due to their fiber, magnesium, and vitamin B6 content. I also opted for okra instead of celery because it has more fiber, magnesium, vitamin B6, and vitamin A. The beans in this recipe replace the sausage that is usually in traditional jambalaya. I'm not a big proponent of vegan sausage since it's processed, but it could be fun in this recipe on occasion, especially if you are serving a crowd!

Heat the avocado oil in a large pot over medium heat. Add the onion and sauté until it turns translucent, 4–5 minutes. Stir in the bell pepper, parsnip, and okra and cook, stirring occasionally for 5–7 minutes.

Stir in the thyme, oregano, paprika, onion powder, sea salt, black pepper, and cayenne pepper. Cook for 1 minute, then add the brown rice, vegetable broth, crushed tomatoes, tamari, and bay leaves. Bring to a boil. Stir in the kidney beans and cannellini beans. Cover and reduce the heat to simmer, stirring occasionally, for 40–45 minutes, or until the rice is cooked.

To serve, divide the stew among bowls and top with any optional toppings. Store in an airtight container in the refrigerator for up to 4 days.

SERVES: 4–5

2 tablespoons avocado oil

½ white onion, chopped

1 bell pepper, chopped

1 parsnip, chopped

1 cup sliced okra, fresh or frozen and thawed (or celery)

1 teaspoon dried thyme

1 teaspoon dried oregano

1 teaspoon smoked paprika

1 teaspoon onion powder

½ teaspoon sea salt

½ teaspoon black pepper

½ teaspoon ground cayenne pepper

1 cup uncooked brown rice

3 cups low-sodium vegetable broth

1 (14-ounce) can crushed tomatoes

2 tablespoons tamari

2 bay leaves

1 (15-ounce) can kidney beans, drained and rinsed

1 (15-ounce) can cannellini beans, drained and rinsed

Optional toppings: fresh parsley, green onions, hot sauce

Buffalo Chickpea Tacos with Hemp Ranch

SERVES: 3–4

TACOS

1 ½ teaspoons avocado oil

¼ red onion, chopped

2 (15-ounce) cans chickpeas, drained and rinsed

½ zucchini, chopped small

½ cup vegan buffalo sauce, homemade (see below) or store-bought

8 10-inch gluten-free tortillas of your choice

2 cups spinach or chopped kale

Optional Toppings: red onion, cilantro, shredded cabbage

HOMEMADE BUFFALO SAUCE

½ cup hot sauce

¼ cup melted vegan butter (I like Earth Balance)

1 tablespoon white vinegar

1 ½ teaspoons paprika

¼ teaspoon garlic powder

VEGAN HEMP RANCH

½ cup filtered water

2 tablespoons olive oil

1 ½ tablespoons white vinegar

⅓ cup hemp hearts

⅓ cup raw cashews, soaked in hot water for 10 minutes, then drained and rinsed

2 chopped green onions

1 clove minced garlic

1 handful fresh parsley

1 teaspoon sea salt

1 teaspoon dried dill

I don't know about you, but once in a while, I just CRAVE buffalo sauce. These tacos are super quick for nights when you don't have a lot of time. The secret is, of course, the sauce. You can follow my recipe for homemade buffalo sauce or buy it at the store to save time (just make sure it's vegan). The easy Vegan Hemp Ranch brings a nice creamy and cooling contrast to the spicy heat of the sauce, and you can make it ahead of time to keep on hand. The chickpeas are high in protein, fiber, iron, magnesium, vitamin B6, and calcium for a filling meal. Use tortillas of your choice, and feel free to add in your favorite veggies alongside the zucchini and spinach.

If making your own buffalo sauce, combine all the ingredients for the sauce in a small bowl or jar and whisk to combine. Set aside.

Combine all the ingredients for the Vegan Hemp Ranch in a small blender and blend until smooth. Set aside.

Heat the avocado oil in a medium sauté pan over medium-high heat. Add the red onion and sauté until it turns translucent, 4–5 minutes. Stir in the chickpeas, zucchini, and buffalo sauce, reduce the heat to medium-low, and cook for 7–10 minutes, or until the sauce has slightly reduced. Turn off the heat.

To assemble each taco, fill a tortilla with some of the spinach, buffalo chickpeas, and hemp ranch, and add additional desired toppings. Serve immediately. Store leftovers in an airtight container in the refrigerator for up to 3 days.

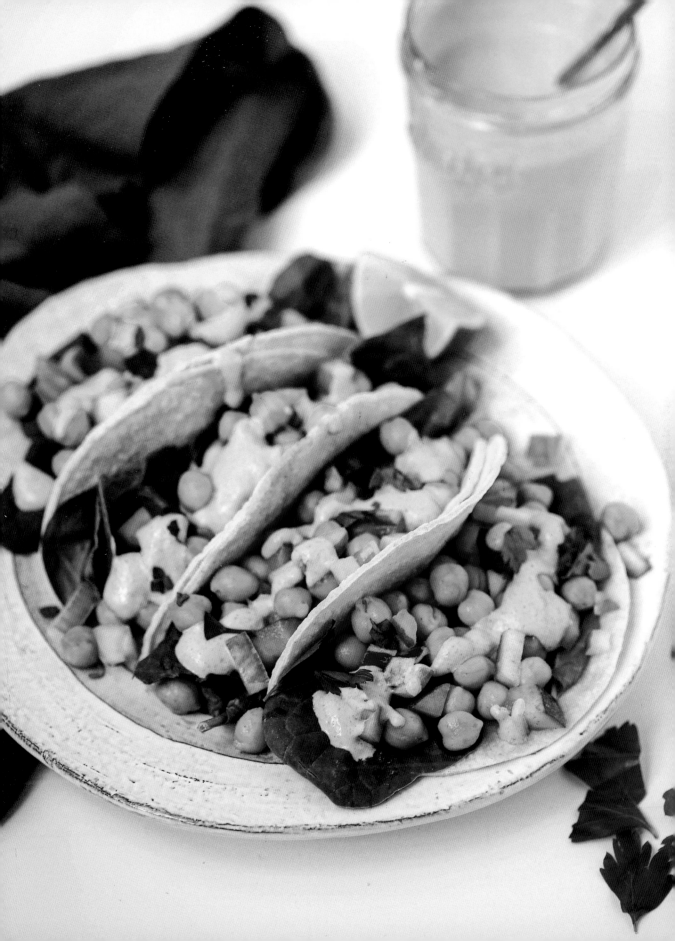

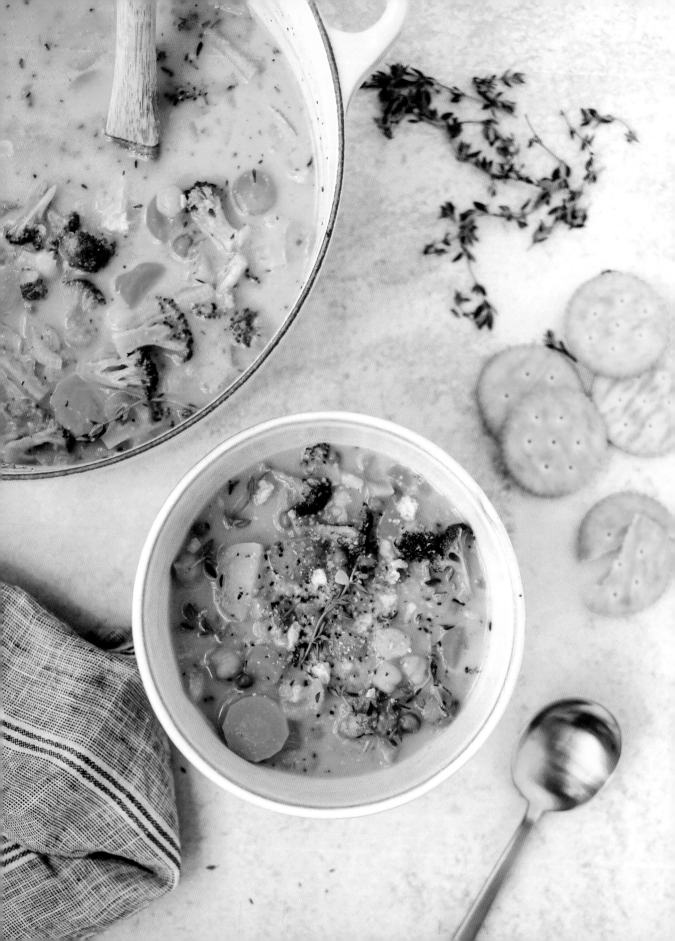

Chickpea Pot Pie Soup

Pot pie might be the ultimate comfort food—and here you can enjoy those cozy flavors in soup form! This is a high-veggie one-pot meal that is lick-the-bowl-clean delicious. You get the creamy consistency by adding a little bit of canned coconut milk and pureeing a portion of the soup. The celery, carrots, gold potatoes, broccoli, peas, and chickpeas pack in plenty of fiber and protein, making it filling and nourishing. You can also add kale for extra greens.

Heat the avocado oil in a large pot over medium heat. Add the onion and sauté for 4–5 minutes, or until translucent. Stir in the celery, carrots, potatoes, garlic, thyme, sea salt, and black pepper. Sauté for 5–6 minutes to soften slightly.

Add the broccoli, chickpeas, vegetable broth, and coconut milk. Bring to a boil, then reduce the heat to simmer, slightly covered, for 15 minutes, or until the potatoes are fork-tender.

Remove 1 cup of potatoes and 1 cup of the liquid (try not to remove any broccoli, unless you want the soup to turn green!). Transfer to a blender and blend until smooth (careful, it's very hot!), or use a hand immersion blender to blend in a large bowl until creamy. Transfer the pureed mixture back to the pot and stir. Mix in the peas and allow the soup to simmer for 5–10 more minutes. Turn off the heat and stir in the lemon juice.

Do a taste test and add more salt and black pepper, if needed. To serve, divide the soup among four bowls and garnish with thyme or black pepper. Serve with crackers or a side salad. Store leftovers in an airtight container in the refrigerator for up to 3 days, or freeze for up to 2 months.

SERVES: 4

2 tablespoons avocado oil

½ yellow onion, chopped

3 stalks celery, chopped

3 large carrots, sliced

2 cups Yukon gold potatoes, cubed

1 clove garlic, minced

1 teaspoon dried thyme, plus more to garnish

1 teaspoon sea salt, plus more as needed

1 teaspoon black pepper, plus more as needed

3 cups broccoli florets

1 (15-ounce) can chickpeas, drained and rinsed

2 cups low-sodium vegetable broth

1 ½ cups canned light coconut milk

1 cup frozen peas

Juice of ½ lemon

"Cheesy" Potato Nachos

SERVES: 2–3

NACHOS

2 russet potatoes, peeled and sliced into ¼- to ½-inch-thick rounds (I use a mandoline slicer)

1 tablespoon avocado oil

Pinch of sea salt

2 cups romaine or kale (optional)

Optional toppings: guacamole, refried beans, black beans, white beans, corn, salsa, pico de gallo, red onion, cilantro, lime juice, crushed tortilla chips

CHEESE SAUCE

½ cup cashews

½ cup nutritional yeast

½ cup filtered water

1 tablespoon fresh lemon juice

¼ teaspoon sea salt

¼ teaspoon ground turmeric

¼ teaspoon onion powder

Pinch of smoked paprika

These nachos hit the spot (especially if you're PMSing!). You may think it's impossible, but you CAN make nachos a healthy way! The first step is baking potato slices to a crisp with high-heat avocado oil instead of frying them. And instead of using a processed fake cheese sauce, we'll make our own vegan cheese sauce that is much healthier and super simple. From there, you can choose whatever toppings your plant-based heart desires—guacamole, refried beans, black beans, pico de gallo, red onion, cilantro, you name it. I like to arrange the crispy potatoes over a bed of lettuce or kale, but feel free to serve plain or with a side salad instead.

Preheat the oven to 375°F. Line a baking sheet with parchment paper.

Toss the potatoes with the avocado oil and sea salt in a large bowl. Arrange the potatoes on the lined baking sheet. It's okay if some of them overlap. Bake the potatoes for 20 minutes, then flip and bake for 15–20 more minutes, or until lightly browned.

While the potatoes bake, soak the cashews for the cheese sauce in hot water for 10 minutes, then drain and rinse. Combine the cashews and other ingredients for the cheese sauce in a small blender and blend until smooth and creamy. Set aside.

Arrange a bed of lettuce or kale on a large plate, if using, then arrange the potato rounds in a pile. Drizzle the cheese sauce over the top (save any remaining cheese sauce for topping other meals), finish with any optional toppings, and serve immediately. Potatoes may become soggy if stored as leftovers.

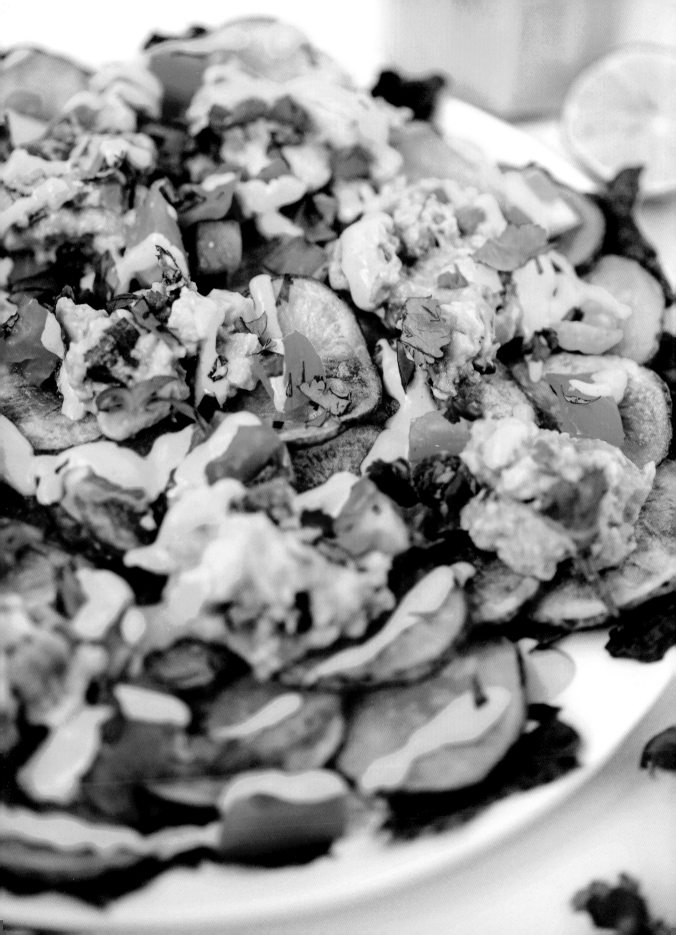

Spicy Squash Enchiladas with White "Queso"

SERVES: 4–5

ENCHILADAS

1 tablespoon avocado oil

½ red onion, chopped

1 small bell pepper, chopped

1 clove garlic, minced

1 jalapeño, chopped (optional)

3 cups peeled and cubed butternut squash (1 small squash)

2 teaspoons ground cumin

2 teaspoons chili powder

1 teaspoon paprika

¼ teaspoon sea salt

⅓ cup filtered water

1 (15-ounce) can cannellini beans, drained and rinsed

1 (15-ounce) jar enchilada sauce, divided

10 (6-inch) corn tortillas (or gluten-free tortillas of your choice)

Optional toppings: cilantro, avocado, hot sauce

The vegan white queso in these enchiladas is addicting, and you can use it for other recipes, too—try it in tacos, dips, and nachos. Yum! While I generally don't recommend store-bought sauces, I used pre-made enchilada sauce here to save time since this recipe has a fair amount of steps already (totally worth it, I promise!). I found a clean one by the Siete brand that was super tasty. Enchiladas are typically made with black beans, but I went with cannellini beans and butternut squash to make these phase-friendly and for added protein and fiber.

Preheat the oven to 350°F. Spray a 13x9-inch baking pan with nonstick cooking spray, or grease with avocado oil.

Heat the avocado oil in a large skillet over medium heat. Add the red onion and sauté for 4–5 minutes, or until translucent. Add the bell pepper, garlic, and jalapeño, if using. Cook for 2 minutes, then add the butternut squash, cumin, chili powder, paprika, and sea salt and mix.

Pour in the water, stir, and cover to steam cook, stirring occasionally, for about 8 minutes or until fork-tender. Add more water if needed so the squash doesn't burn. Once the squash is fork-tender, turn off the heat. Stir in the cannellini beans and ½ cup of the enchilada sauce.

To assemble the enchiladas, pour about ⅓ cup of enchilada sauce into the prepared pan and spread it around to make an even layer. Wrap the tortillas in a wet paper towel and microwave them for 20–30 seconds (this makes rolling easier).

Spoon ⅓ cup of the squash filling into each tortilla, then roll and place seam side down in the baking pan. Pour the remaining enchilada sauce over the top. Bake for 25 minutes.

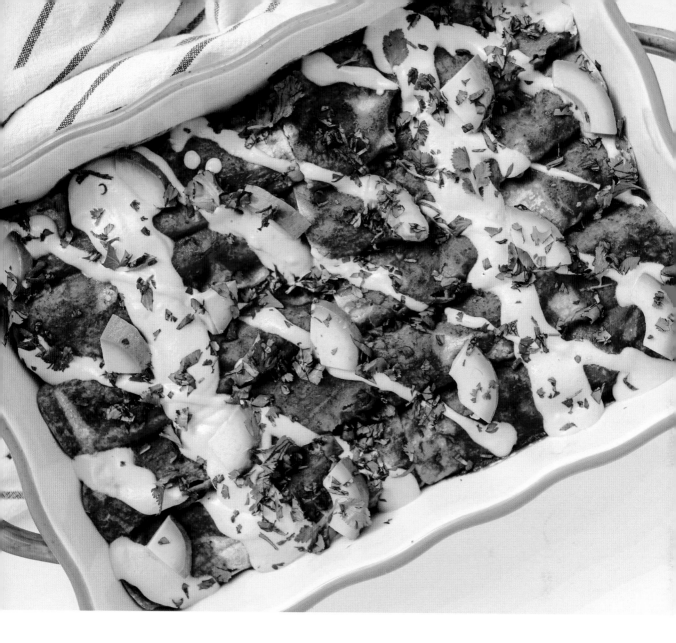

Meanwhile, make the White Queso. Combine all the ingredients for the queso in a small blender and blend until smooth. If it's too thick, add 1–2 tablespoons more water to reach the desired consistency. Set aside.

Once the enchiladas are done baking, remove from the oven and drizzle the white queso over the top. Sprinkle with any optional toppings and serve. Store leftovers in an airtight container in the refrigerator for up to 3 days.

WHITE "QUESO"

½ cup cashews, soaked in hot water for 10 minutes, then drained and rinsed

1 (4-ounce) can diced green chiles

⅓ cup nutritional yeast

¼ cup filtered water

1 ½ teaspoons fresh lemon juice (or apple cider vinegar)

¼ teaspoon sea salt

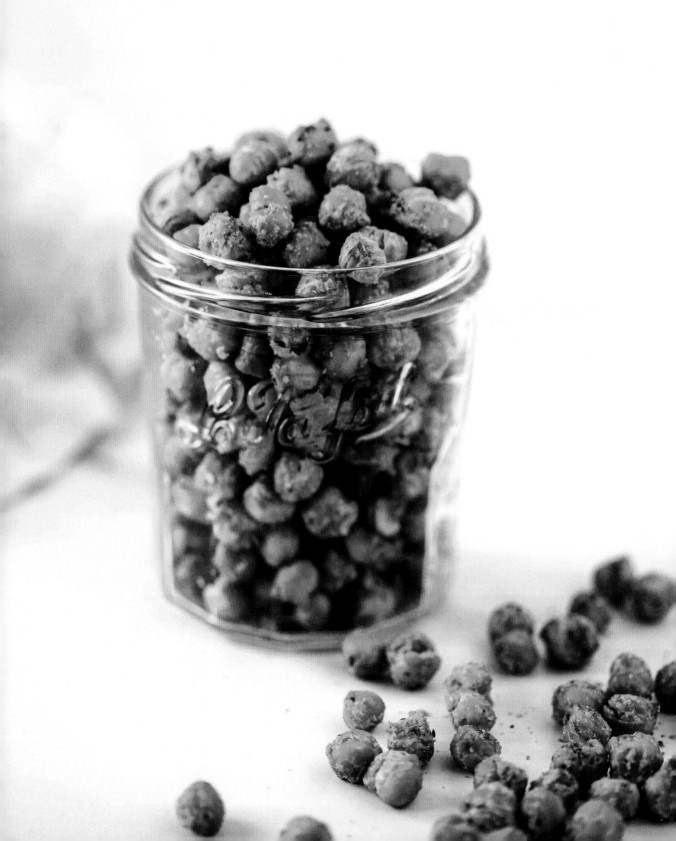

Prep Time: 10 minutes   **Cook Time:** 50 minutes   **Total Time:** 60 minutes

Spicy "Honey" Mustard–Roasted Chickpeas

I love anything with a honey mustard flavor, but remember, honey is not vegan! In this sweet and spicy snack, we're friendly to the bees by using maple syrup instead. It's essential to keep healthy snacks on hand when trying to balance out your hormones and keep your blood sugar steady. These have a satisfying crunch, and I love to snack on them while working or running errands. Staying away from processed snacks can help calm inflammation in the body and lead to healthier periods. Make a big batch and grab these roasted chickpeas whenever you are in need of a real-food snack.

SERVES: 5–6

2 (15-ounce) cans chickpeas, drained and rinsed (see Note)

2 tablespoons avocado oil

2 tablespoons yellow mustard

1–2 tablespoons pure maple syrup

¾ teaspoon sea salt

½ teaspoon ground cayenne pepper

½ teaspoon onion powder

½ teaspoon black pepper

Preheat the oven to 400°F. Line a baking sheet with parchment paper.

Combine all the ingredients in a medium mixing bowl, beginning with 1 tablespoon of the maple syrup and adding more as needed to reach your desired sweetness level. Mix well, making sure all the chickpeas are evenly coated.

Transfer the chickpeas to the baking sheet and spread them out evenly. Bake for 25 minutes, mix around, then bake for another 20–25 minutes, or until the chickpeas are golden and crispy.

Let cool for 5 minutes. Store leftovers in an airtight container at room temperature, or in the refrigerator for up to 4 days.

Note: For extra-crispy chickpeas, the trick is to remove the chickpea "skins" before adding the spices. This is a time-consuming step, but it works!

Chickpea Flatbread

MAKES: 4-5 FLATBREADS

1 cup chickpea flour

1 cup filtered water

½ teaspoon sea salt

1 tablespoon coconut oil

These flatbreads are so fun and simple to make—they only have three ingredients! Think of them as a pancake's savory cousin. They are the perfect snack for dipping or pairing with a soup or stew. I like to eat them with Pumpkin Hummus (on the next page). Spread some hummus on them and roll them up and eat them—bonus points for adding some cucumber, celery, or carrots. This recipe calls for chickpea flour, which is easy to find at a store similar to Whole Foods or online.

Combine the chickpea flour, water, and sea salt in a medium mixing bowl. Whisk together. The batter will be very thin, and there may be a few small clumps.

Heat the coconut oil in a large skillet over medium heat. Once hot, pour the batter into the skillet as if you were cooking pancakes, one at a time. The batter is thin, so it will spread a lot. You can make them whatever size you want.

Cook the flatbread for 3–4 minutes, or until you see bubbles forming on the whole surface of the flatbread. Flip and cook the other side for 3–4 minutes, then transfer to a plate. Repeat with the remaining batter, adding additional coconut oil as needed between flatbreads to prevent sticking.

Serve the flatbreads immediately with hummus or your favorite dip. Wrap leftovers in aluminum foil in the refrigerator for up to 2 days.

Pumpkin Hummus

There are so many hummus recipes out there that I debated even putting one in the book, but this one was too perfect for the luteal phase not to include. It combines chickpeas, tahini, and—the star of the show—pumpkin puree, which gives it an even smoother creamy texture and extra phase-friendly nutrients. I love pairing it with veggies or the Chickpea Flatbread.

Combine all the ingredients in a food processor. Blend/pulse until smooth and creamy, scraping down the sides a few times as needed. If it seems too thick, you can add 1–2 tablespoons of water to reach the desired consistency. Taste and adjust the amount of sea salt, lemon, and cayenne pepper as needed.

Transfer the pumpkin hummus to a serving bowl, garnish with a drizzle of olive oil, and sprinkle with optional toppings as desired. Serve with veggies, Chickpea Flatbreads, or pita for dipping. Store any leftovers in an airtight container in the refrigerator for up to 4 days.

SERVES: 3–4

1 (15-ounce) can chickpeas, drained and rinsed

½ cup pumpkin puree (not pumpkin pie filling)

3 tablespoons tahini

2 tablespoons olive oil

Juice of 1 lemon, or more as needed

½ teaspoon ground cumin

½ teaspoon paprika

½ teaspoon sea salt, or more as needed

¼ teaspoon ground cayenne pepper, or more as needed

Optional Toppings: olive oil, paprika, parsley, sesame seeds

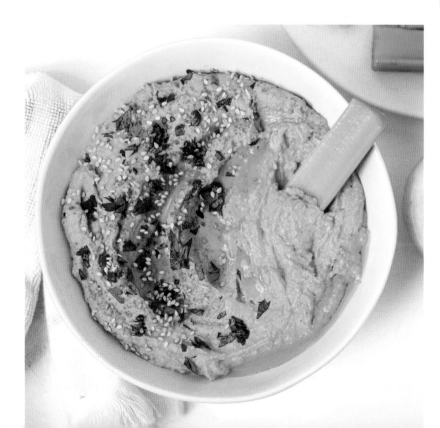

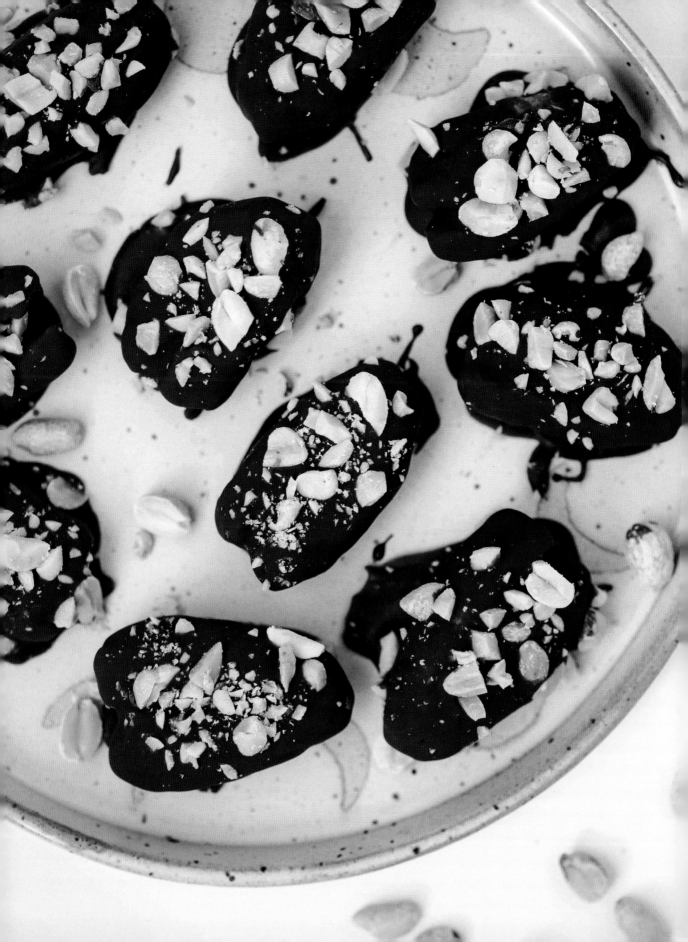

Prep Time: 10 minutes   **Freeze Time:** 30 minutes   **Total Time:** 40 minutes

Healthy "Snickers" Bites

Say hello to your new favorite treat, inspired by the classic Snickers candy bar. They're essentially peanut butter-stuffed dates dunked in melted vegan chocolate and sprinkled with chopped peanuts. These are a must-have for those chocolate cravings during your luteal phase. And did you know that it makes sense to crave chocolate while PMSing? Dark chocolate, in particular, is high in magnesium, which helps calm our nervous system, reduce cortisol, support our mood, and relax sore muscles or cramping in the uterus. See, your body knows what it's doing! The medjool dates are high in fiber and taste like caramel. Dreamy, right?

MAKES: 10 BITES

10 medjool dates

⅓ cup peanut butter (or any nut or seed butter)

½ cup vegan chocolate chips (preferably dark chocolate)

1 teaspoon coconut oil

3 tablespoons chopped peanuts (or any nuts or seeds)

Line a baking sheet or plate with parchment paper. Gently open up each date to remove the pit, but don't rip it in half; you want it to still hold together somewhat. Stuff about ½ tablespoon of peanut butter into each date and lay them flat on the lined baking sheet.

Combine the vegan chocolate chips and coconut oil in a small microwave-safe bowl. Heat in the microwave in 30-second increments, stirring in between to prevent burning, until fully melted.

Drop a stuffed date into the melted chocolate and use a fork to roll it around, making sure it's well coated in chocolate. Place the chocolate-covered date back on the parchment paper and sprinkle with some of the chopped peanuts. Repeat with all the remaining dates.

Place the baking sheet or plate in the freezer until the chocolate has set, about 30 minutes (if you can wait that long!). Serve straight from the freezer or allow to thaw for a few minutes.

Store in an airtight container in the refrigerator or freezer to prevent melting for up to 2 weeks.

Banana Bonbons

MAKES: 8–10 BONBONS

2 ripe bananas, sliced thick into rounds

½ cup vegan chocolate chips

1 ½ teaspoons coconut oil

Optional toppings: cacao nibs, shredded coconut, flaky sea salt, ground cinnamon, chia seeds

In these bite-sized treats, creamy bananas are smothered in melted chocolate and kissed with cacao nibs, coconut, flaky sea salt, cinnamon, and chia seeds. Is your mouth watering yet? To make these even more decadent, drizzle some almond butter over the chocolate. I like to keep these in the freezer to plan ahead AND because the chocolate has a nice crunch when it's frozen. Bananas are sweet, high in fiber, and a great source of Vitamin B6, which can help decrease the PMS symptoms that are all too common in the luteal phase. So, eat your bananas . . . I mean, your chocolate-covered bananas!

Line a baking sheet or plate with parchment paper. Lay the banana slices flat on the sheet.

Combine the vegan chocolate chips and coconut oil in a small microwave-safe bowl. Heat in the microwave in 30-second increments, stirring in between to prevent burning, until fully melted.

Drop a banana slice into the melted chocolate and use a fork to roll it around, making sure it's well coated in chocolate. Place the chocolate-covered banana back on the parchment paper and sprinkle with any of the optional toppings. Repeat with the remaining banana slices.

Place the baking sheet or plate in the freezer until the chocolate has set, about 30 minutes. Serve straight from the freezer or allow to thaw for a few minutes. Store in an airtight container in the freezer for up to 2 months.